MEETING MENTAL HEALTH NEEDS

SERVICE DELIVERY IN ISRAEL

MENTAL ILLNESSES AND TREATMENTS

Additional books in this series can be found on Nova's website
under the Series tab.

Additional e-books in this series can be found on Nova's website
under the e-book tab.

MEETING MENTAL HEALTH NEEDS

SERVICE DELIVERY IN ISRAEL

ALEXANDER M. PONIZOVSKY, M.D., PH.D.
AND
ALEXANDER GRINSHPOON, M.D., PH.D.

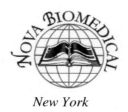

New York

Library of Congress Cataloging-in-Publication Data

ISBN: 978-1-63117-306-6

Library of Congress Control Number: 2014931905

Published by Nova Science Publishers, Inc. † New York

CONTENTS

PREFACE

This book summarizes findings of the authors' studies that are united by a common theme of needs of psychiatric patients in Israel. The studies were carried out during the past decade, during the period when the second author, Prof. Alexander Grinshpoon was the Head of Mental Health Services in the Ministry of Health (2001-2006), and later in collaboration with the Research Unit of Mental Health Services where the first author, Dr. Alexander Ponizovsky, is employed. We were motivated by our own need to learn more about met and mainly unmet needs of people with mental disorders. This knowledge was not a goal, but rather an urgent prerequisite for developing innovative health services or adjusting the existing ones to meet the needs and increase both quality of care and quality of life of our patients. Although the conception of need is composite and can be defined in multiple ways to include different aspects of common desires that motivate human activities and ways of their fulfillment, for our purposes, we accepted the Bradshaw definition of need (1972) as 'perceived' need or what individuals believe they require. Within the context of health care, a need was considered a lack of health or welfare, or insufficient access to care. All of the investigations paralleled the Mental Health Reform in Israel. During this period the structural reform was implemented and reduction of hospital beds and development of community based facilities were initiated. The studies therefore, reflect the specific needs and demands of deinstitutionalization. In Israel, the second stage of the reform is currently in progress as the responsibility for mental health care is being transferred to the health funds, which now handle all aspects of both physical and mental health care.

The selection of topics, the emphasis on briefly summarizing research findings rather than exhaustively reviewing the scientific literature and providing practical recommendations are intended to make the book an interesting and useful resource for policymakers, clinicians, and other health professionals, such as clinical psychologists, social workers, occupational therapists, general and family medical practitioners, nursing personnel, family members and other support persons, and perhaps persons with mental disorders and their families and caregivers.

The book includes ten chapters. All focus on fulfilling the needs of mental health patients. The first three chapters introduce the reader to the problem of needs, definitions and methods of their assessment, and familiarize readers with our findings of our research on the needs of psychiatric patients in Israel. Chapters four and five describe a variety of psychiatric care and rehabilitation services in Israel and the reform in the psychiatric service delivery system. It also covers research findings regarding the consequences of the massive deinstitutionalization, survival of the former psychiatric residents in the community settings and the problem of re-institutionalization as a rebound phenomenon. Chapter six addresses the issues of traditional forensic psychiatric services (involuntary hospitalization, forensic psychiatric evaluation) and new forms, for example, legal representation of involuntarily hospitalized patients before the District Psychiatric Board for discharge. Chapters seven and eight focus on the need for mental health services among ethnic groups; needs for service utilization under terrorism. Chapter nine describes a novel service developed for psychiatric emergency needs, and chapter ten presents an assessment of oral and dental health needs of institutionalized patients and improved dental services delivery, as part of the rehabilitation and enhancement of self-esteem of the patients. Each chapter suggests practical applications for fulfilling the specific needs of the population of individuals with mental disorders and can be useful for a wide circle of mental health professionals. The book is an example of the integration of research and administration policies that oversee implementation of the study findings to improve mental health services.

ACKNOWLEDGMENTS

Our sincere appreciation is expressed to the entire staff of the Department of Mental Health Services, Israel Ministry of Health, for cooperation in all aspects of our research whose goal is to improve the quality of life of the population of individuals with mental disorders. The staff also assisted in implementation of the research findings, for the benefit of our patients. Special thanks to the staff of the District Psychiatrists, and to the Division of Dental Health, Israel Ministry of Health.

We would like to thank Rena Kurs, medical librarian at Sha'ar Menashe Mental Health Center, for her assistance in the preparation and language editing of this book.

And finally, we'd like to thank our families and loved ones for their gracious support and patience during the long hours it took to produce this book.

Dr. A.M. Ponizovsky was supported in part by the Ministry of Immigrant Absorption.

Chapter 1

IDENTIFICATION OF NEEDS AMONG PATIENTS WITH SEVERE MENTAL ILLNESS

ABSTRACT

Schizophrenia, perhaps the most severe mental illness (SMI), is a chronic psychiatric disorder characterized by disruptive and distressing positive and negative symptoms, and cognitive impairments. The consequences of SMIs are often translated into unmet needs. Although there is consensus among mental health policymakers, providers and clinicians that mental health services should be provided on the basis of need, the concept of client needs is equivocal and varies substantially among professionals, patients and involved family care providers. In this chapter, the concept of met and unmet needs of patients with SMI is presented and key concepts are defined. Given the importance of studying needs of patients with SMI from the policymaker's perspective, the background for a study performed by the authors to examine and compare the perception of needs by staff, patients and their families and the relationship of unmet needs to clinical symptoms, distress and quality of life is presented. The chapter concludes with the delineation of the research hypotheses.

INTRODUCTION

Schizophrenia is a complex and perhaps the most severe mental illness. It is a chronic psychiatric disorder that adversely affects a broad range of psychological processes and is characterized by a constellation of distinctive and recognizable symptoms (Andreasen and Olsen, 1982; Schultz and

Andreasen, 1999; Mueser and McGurk, 2004). Schizophrenia symptomatology is traditionally divided into positive symptoms, typified by grossly abnormal behavior such as delusions, hallucinations, and thought disturbances and 'negative' or 'deficit' symptoms that are less obvious but equally serious. Negative symptoms represent the absence of normal behavior and include flat or blunted affect (i.e., lack of emotional expression, apathy, and social withdrawal), an inability to start and follow through with activities, alogia, poverty of speech, and social withdrawal that leads to lack of pleasure or interest in life. Although the positive-negative dichotomy is a simplification because it does not cover the entire spectrum of schizophrenic psychopathology (e.g., cognitive impairments), it has important clinical and prognostic significance. While positive symptoms are preponderant at the onset of illness or during phases of acute exacerbation and are often ameliorated with antipsychotic drug therapy, negative symptoms generally appear during the chronic deteriorating course and are generally treatment-resistant (even with novel antipsychotic agents). Negative symptoms account for the bulk of disability caused by the disease.

The clinical symptoms of schizophrenia and other severe mental illnesses (schizoaffective and bipolar disorders) are often disruptive and distressing. Their consequences that are often translated to unmet needs are no less severe—truncated education, unemployment, social isolation, and exclusion from the general community.

Needs have been defined as "the requirements of individuals to enable them to achieve, maintain or restore an acceptable level of social independence or quality of life" (Department of Health Social Services Inspectorate, 1991). It is especially important to understand the needs of individuals with serious mental disorders that often manifest in social and personal disadvantages, in order to initiate appropriate interventions to improve their quality of life (Werner, 2011).

Although there is consensus among mental health policymakers, providers and clinicians, that mental health services should be provided on the basis of need (Lasalvia et al., 2000a), the concept of client needs is equivocal and varies substantially among professionals, patients and involved family care providers.

Using the Camberwell Assessment of Need (CAN), Grinshpoon and colleagues (2008) surveyed 52 inpatients with schizophrenia and schizoaffective disorders in order to identify their needs and compare them with needs as rated by the nursing staff and patients' relatives. Findings revealed significant differences in the perceptions of the patients and staff in six of the 22 CAN domains. Patients rated the needs for "information on condition and treatment" and "benefits" higher, while the staff gave higher ratings to the patients' needs for "intimate relationships", "safety for others", "self-care" and "daytime activities". Differences were also revealed between the patients and their relatives in the same need areas. Recently, Werner (2011) found that care providers reported a higher number of met needs, and patients reported more unmet needs and more areas in which there were no perceived needs, suggesting that the distinction between no needs and met needs is also difficult to make.

The investigation of needs as determined by patients and providers is important for two reasons. First, needs have direct implications for treatment and should be the premise for care planning. Second, accumulating evidence indicates that actual unmet and met needs better predict patients' quality of life than either their clinical characteristics (symptomatology, diagnosis) or socio-demographic characteristics (Hansson et al., 2003; Slade et al., 2005, Werner, 2011). Moreover, evidence has accumulated regarding an association between patient's needs and satisfaction with the care they receive (Leese et al. 1998 Gerson and Rose, 2012) and some aspects of staff-rated social disability (Issakidis and Teesson 1999; Slade et al., 1999a; Lasalvia et al., 2008). In addition, comparing assessments of needs from different perspectives provides a powerful means of patient evaluation and is potentially valuable information for care planning (Grinshpoon et al., 2008). Facing multiple severe life stressors with minimal resources, people with severe mental illnesses often require a variety of support services to fulfill their major subjective as well as objective needs such as adequate income, meaningful employment, decent and affordable housing, quality health care, and education to optimize skills (Ball and Havassy, 1984). If needs are to be the basis of the care provided for patients who utilize psychiatric services, it is an important aim to develop a better understanding of the profiles of patients with unmet needs, for use both in service planning and in providing the highest quality of care. With this goal in mind, we present a multi-axial approach to identifying the correlates of high-need patients.

THE CONCEPT OF NEED

The concept of need originated with Maslow, who set out a hierarchy of universal needs as a model for understanding human actions (Maslow, 1954). He proposed that people are motivated by the requirement to fulfill these needs, and that higher needs (e.g., need for friends) could be met once lower and more fundamental needs (e.g., need for food) had been met.

In psychiatry, the concept of need can be used in various ways to express the relationship between psychiatric disorders, the behavior of those suffering from the disorder and the response of those whose task it is to alleviate the discomfort. Brewin et al (1987) defined a need as present when a person's level of functioning falls below, or threatens to fall below, some specified level, and when there is some remediable, or potentially remediable, cause. Bradshaw (1972) proposed the following taxonomy of needs:

- 'perceived' need — what individuals believe they require
- 'expressed' need — the demand for services represented by utilization data
- 'comparative' need — arises from comparison with other groups or individuals
- 'normative' need — need as defined by professionals (experts)

The simplest definition of normative need is the capacity to benefit from treatment or care. Needs are defined in terms of problems for which 'state-of-the-art' solutions exist. The fact that needs are identified does not mean they will be met. For instance, a professionally defined need may remain unmet or replaced by one lower in the hierarchy, simply because the user does not acknowledge the defined need.

Given the importance of studying needs of patients with SMI from the policymaker's perspective, Grinshpoon et al (2008a,b) performed a study to examine and compare:

- the need profiles, at group levels, of hospitalized patients with SMI
- staff, patients' and patients' families' and friends' perceptions of patients' needs
- the relationship between patients' needs and their socio-demographic and clinical variables and quality of life

The authors examined the met and unmet needs of mentally ill inpatients and addressed the following research questions:

- How do schizophrenia patients perceive their met and unmet needs?

- How does the nursing staff on psychiatric wards perceive schizophrenia patients' met and unmet needs?
- How do schizophrenia patients' relatives and friends perceive the patients' met and unmet needs?
- What is the difference in the perception of unmet needs between schizophrenia patients and their schizoaffective counterparts?
- What is the relationship between unmet needs and the socio-demographic characteristics of these patients?
- What is the relationship among unmet needs, levels of distress, clinical symptoms and characteristics, and quality of life and functioning?

To facilitate further discussion of these questions, theoretical and operational definitions of the study terms are provided here.

Needs

Theoretically, we used Bradshaw's definition of 'perceived' need or what individuals believe they require. Within the context of health care, we used Brewin's definition of need as a lack of health or welfare, or a lack of access to care. Operationally, the Camberwell Assessment of Need was used to determine patient's needs (CAN-R; Slade et al., 1996). Ponizovsky et al (2013) examined the agreement between the Camberwell Assessment of Need Short Appraisal Schedule self-report version (CANSAS-P) and the Camberwell Assessment of Need (CAN) interview-based scale in 100 outpatients with schizophrenia and schizoaffective disorders. In line with previous studies, they found high agreement between the two instruments that supports the inter-changeability of CANSAS-P and CAN. Given that CANSAS-P use is more economical and quicker to administer than the CAN, it was determined that it can be used as a reliable screening tool to detect care needs among patients with schizophrenia and schizoaffective disorders.

Quality of Life

Theoretically, subjective quality of life (QOL) is considered a non-specific perception of an individual's total existence (Lehman, 1983; Headley et al.,

1993; Oliver et al., 1996), the assessment of which serves as an indicator of subjective wellbeing (Horley, 1984; Bech et al., 2001; Ruggeri et al., 2001). Most conceptualizations of health-related QOL include the dimensions of physical, social, and role functioning, mental health, and general health perceptions, including concepts such as energy, fatigue, pain, and cognitive functioning (Wilson and Cleary, 1995). These physical, psychological, and social domains of health are seen as distinct areas influenced by a person's experiences, beliefs, expectations, and perceptions (Testa and Simonson, 1996). Indeed, psychiatric symptoms have been reported to have only a limited relationship with QOL in schizophrenia, while psychosocial effects of mental illness (e.g., social support, self-esteem, and self-efficacy) were found to have a greater impact on QOL (Ritsner, 2003; Werner, 2012).Operationally, while there is no universally accepted definition of QOL, most investigators agree that patients' statements on satisfaction with major life domains of daily functioning are relevant indicators of subjective QOL (WHO QOL Group, 1995; Lehman, 1996; Priebe et al., 2000). The patient's total score on the Global Life Functioning inventory (Elkin et al., 1985) and on its general wellbeing and functioning subscales (Pedersen et al., 2002), was used to operationally define patients' QOL, with higher scores indicating better outcomes.

Psychological distress. Theoretically, psychological distress was defined as the reaction of an individual to external or internal stresses, characterized by a mixture of psychological symptoms, such as poor self-esteem, hopelessness, helplessness, dread, confused thinking, sadness, anxiety, and psycho-physiological symptoms (Dohrenwend et al., 1980). *These nonspecific responses to stressful events vary in intensity, and constitute proxy measures of mild to severe psychopathology. If the extent to which these symptoms are expressed was not sufficient to diagnose a specific mental disorder according to ICD or DSM criteria, they were diagnosed as psychological distress or, sometimes, as demoralization syndrome.* Operationally, psychological distress was defined as the patient's total score on the General Health Questionnaire (Goldberg and Williams, 1988), with higher scores indicating more intensive distress.

Clinical symptoms. Theoretically, researchers have shown that both the positive and the negative symptom domains are important in predicting clinical, economic and social outcomes for schizophrenia patients (Revicki et al., 1996; Perlick et al., 1999). Furthermore, the severity of these symptoms directly impacts the patient's quality of life and inpatient hospitalizations.

A three-factor model of schizophrenia includes a third symptom grouping, the 'disorganization syndrome'. This distinction places thought disorder and related disorganized behavior in a separate symptom cluster from delusions and hallucinations. A five-factor model comprises five symptom dimensions — positive, negative, disorganized, affective, and excited (Kay and Sevy, 1990). Operationally, clinical symptoms of schizophrenia were defined as the patient's total score on the Positive and Negative Syndrome Scale (PANSS; Kay et al., 1987) as well as on scores according to the three-factor and pentagonal models (Kay and Sevy, 1990).

The study was based on the premise that schizophrenia patients have prevalent needs for care that may vary and change, but are predictable. The course and duration of chronic illness, as well as higher levels of dysfunction and psychiatric symptoms, are associated with higher levels of unmet needs. Since needs are to a certain extent modifiable, they are amenable to treatment or mental health interventions. The recognition of needs and their socio-demographic, clinical and psychosocial correlates may serve as a basis for the allocation of resources and the delivery of services.

Research Hypotheses

Drawing on the relevant literature, three hypotheses were generated for empirical analysis:

- Staff and family assessments of patients' unmet needs would be higher than the patient's assessments.
- Unmet needs would be higher among those with higher levels of distress and also among those with lower levels of wellbeing, functioning and quality of life.
- Unmet needs would be higher among those with higher levels of psychopathological symptoms.

The null hypotheses were that there will be no differences in assessments of unmet needs:

- between the patients, staff and relatives
- between patients with different levels of distress, clinical symptoms, functioning, and quality of life

The results of this study are presented in Chapter 3 after a detailed review of various methods of assessment of needs in Chapter 2. The findings provide a profile of unmet needs for the psychiatric inpatient population and quantification of the amount of help receiving from formal services and informal agents and the degree of satisfaction with the help.

CONCLUSION

Information concerning unmet needs of individuals with severe mental illness contributes to the implementation of more effective interventions and for the optimization of resource allocation, service planning and delivery, and service utilization by patients with severe mental illness.

REFERENCES

Andreasen NC, Olsen S. Negative versus positive schizophrenia: definition and validation. *Arch Gen Psychiatry* 1982;39:789-794.

Ball FL, Havassy BE. A survey of the problems and needs of homeless consumers of acute psychiatric services. *Hosp Community Psychiatry* 1984;35:917-921.

Bech P, Olson LR, Nimeus A. Psychometric scales in suicide risk assessment. In: Wasserman D (ed). *Suicide: An Unnecessary Death*. London, UK: Dunitz, 2001,pp.147-157.

Bradshaw J. A taxonomy of social need. In *Problems and Progress in Medical Care: Essays on Current Research* (G.McLachlan, ed.) (7th Series). London: Oxford University Press, 1972, pp. 71-82.

Brewin CR, Wing JK, Mangen SP, Brugha TS, MacCarthy B. Principles and practice of measuring needs in the long-term mentally ill: the MRC needs for care assessment. *Psychol Med* 1987;17:971-981.

Department of Health Social Services Inspectorate. *Car management and assessment: Practitioners' guide*. London: HMSO, 1991.

Dohrenwend BP, Shrout PE, Egri G, Mendelsohn FS.Nonspecific psychological distress and other dimensions of psychopathology.Measures for use in the general population. *Arch Gen Psychiatry* 1980;37:1229-1236.

Elkin I, Parloff MB, Hadley SW, Autry JH. NIMH Treatment of Depression Collaborative Research Program. Background and research plan. *Arch Gen Psychiatry* 1985;42:305-316.

Gerson LD, Rose LE. Needs of persons with serious mental illness following discharge from inpatient treatment: patient and family views. *Arch Psychiatr Nurs* 2012;26:261-271.

Goldberg DP, Williams P. *A Users Guide to The General Health Questionnaire: GHQ.* Windsor: NFER-NELSON, 1988.

Grinshpoon A, Friger M, Orev E, Shvarts S, Kaplan Z, Abramowitz MZ, Ponizovsky AM. Relative perceptions of the needs of inpatients with schizophrenia and schizoaffective disorders. *Isr J Psychiatry Relat Sci* 2008a;45:201-209.

Grinshpoon A, Ponizovsky AM. The relationships between need profiles, clinical symptoms, functioning and the well-being of inpatients with severe mental disorders. *J Eval Clin Pract* 2008b;14:218-225.

Hansson L, Sandlund M, Bengtsson-Tops A, Bjarnason O, Karlsson H, Mackeprang T, Merinder L, Nilsson L, Sorgaard K, Vinding H, Middelboe T. The relationship of needs and quality of life in persons with schizophrenia living in the community.A Nordic multi-center study. *Nord J Psychiatry* 2003;57:5-11.

Headley BW, Kelley J, Wearing AJ. Dimensions of mental health: life satisfaction, positive affect, anxiety and depression. *Soc Indicat Res* 1993;29:63-82.

Horley J. Life satisfaction, happiness, and morale: two problems with the use of subjective well-being indicators. *Gerontologist* 1984;24:124-127.

Issakidis C, Teesson M. Measurement of need for care: a trial of the Camberwell Assessment of Need and the health of the nation outcome scales. *Aust N Z J Psychiatry* 1999;33:754–759.

Kay SR, Fiszbein A, Opler LA. The Positive and Negative Syndrome Scale (PANSS) for schizophrenia. *Schizophr Bull* 1987;13:261-276.

Kay SR, Sevy S. Pyramidical model of schizophrenia. *Schizophr Bull* 1990;16:537-545.

Lasalvia A, Bonetto C, Tansella M, Stefani B, Ruggeri M. Does staff-patient agreement on needs for care predict a better mental health outcome? A 4-yearfollow-up in a community service. *Psychol Med* 2008;38:123-133.

Lasalvia A, Ruggeri M, Mazzi MA, Dall'Agnola RB. The perception of needs for care in staff and patients in community-based mental health services.The South-Verona Outcome Project 3. *Acta Psychiatr Scand* 2000;102:366-375.

Leese M, Johnson S, Slade M, Parkman S, Kelly F, Phelan M, Thornicroft G. User perspective on needs and satisfaction with mental health services. PRiSM Psychosis Study 8. *Br J Psychiatry* 1998;173:409-415.

Lehman AF. Measures of quality of life among persons with severe and persistent mental disorders. *Soc Psychiatry Psychiatr Epidemiol* 1996;31:78-88.

Lehman AF. The effects of psychiatric symptoms on uality of life assessments among the chronic mentally ill. *Eval Progr Plan* 1983;6:143-151.

Maslow A. *Motivation and Personality*. New York: Harper and Row, 1954.

Mueser KT, McGurk SR. Schizophrenia. *Lancet* 2004;363:2063–2072.

Oliver J, Huxley P, Bridges K. *Quality of Life and Mental Health Services*. London, UK: Routledge, 1996.

Pedersen RD, Pallay AG, Rudolph RL. Can improvement in well-being and functioning be distinguished from depression improvement in antidepressant clinical trials? *Qual Life Res* 2002;11:9-17.

Perlick DA, Rosenheck RA, Clarkin JF, Sirey J, Raue P. Symptoms predicting inpatient service use among patients with bipolar affective disorder. *Psychiatr Serv* 1999;50:806–812.

Ponizovsky AM, Rothstein I, Grinshpoon A. The CANSAS self-report for screening of needs in outpatients with schizophrenia and schizoaffective disorders. *Community Ment Health J* 2013 Dec 12. (Epub ahead of print).

Priebe S, Roeder-Wanner UU, Kaiser W. Quality of life in first-admitted schizophrenia patients: a follow-up study. *Psychol Med* 2000;30:225-230.

Revicki DA, Leidy NK, Howland L. Evaluating the psychometric characteristics of the Psychological General Well-Being Index with a new response scale. *Qual Life Res* 1996;5:419-425.

Ritsner M. Predicting changes in domain-specific quality of life of schizophrenia patients. *J Nerv Ment Dis* 2003;191:287-294.

Ruggeri M, Bisoffi G, Fontecedro L, Warner R. Subjective and objective dimensions of quality of life in psychiatric patients: a factor analytical approach. *Br J Psychiatry* 2001;178:268-275.

Schultz SK and Andreasen NC.Schizophrenia. *Lancet* 1999;353:1425-1430

Slade M, Leese M, Cahill S, Thornicroft G, Kuipers E. Patient-rated mental health needs and quality of life improvement. *Br J Psychiatry* 2005;187:256-261.

Slade M, Leese M, Taylor R, Thornicroft G. The association between needs and quality of life in an epidemio epidemiologically representative sample of people with psychosis. *Acta Psychiatr Scand* 1999;100:49–57.

Slade M, Phelan M, Thornicroft G, Parkman S. The Camberwell Assessment of Need (CAN): Comparison of assessments by staff and patients of the needs of the severely mentally ill. *Soc Psychiatry Psychiatr Epidemiol* 1996;31:109–113.

Testa MA, Simonson DC.Assessment of quality-of-life outcomes. *N Engl J Med* 1996;334:835-840.

Werner S. Subjective well-being, hope, and needs of individuals with serious mental illness. *Psychiatry Res* 2012;196:214-219.

Werner S. Needs Assessment of Individuals with Serious Mental Illness: Can It Help in Promoting Recovery? *Community Ment Health J* 2011 Dec 4. (Epub ahead of print).

WHOQOL Group. TheWorld Health Organization Quality of Life Assessment (WHOQOL): position paper from the World Health Organization. *Soc Sci Med* 1995;41:1403-1409.

Wilson IB, Cleary PD. Linking clinical variables with health-related quality of life. A conceptual model of patient outcomes. *J Am Med Assoc* 1995;273:59-65.

Chapter 2

ASSESSMENT OF NEEDS

ABSTRACT

For individuals with severe mental illness quantification of needs might facilitate service planning and evaluation, and ultimately promote patient recovery. Various approaches to the assessment of needs, such as epidemiological, socio-demographic and service utilization assessments are presented. The importance of evaluation of needs by key informants such as family members and caregivers and the disparities between patient and carer assessments are discussed. A three factor model (Functional disability, Social loneliness and Emotional loneliness) and a five factor model structure (Basic, Social, Functioning, Health, and Service domains) are put forth for the Camberwell Assessment of Need scale. In the analysis of the authors' research, presented in the following chapter, in addition to the tri-dimensional model the authors also used a model of needs based on 5 aggregated problem areas in the CAN that are discussed here. Findings of the studies presented provide further support for the idea that mental health services should involve patients and their relatives when planning and evaluating psychiatric intervention. This involvement is the basis for developing a partnership care model.

APPROACHES TO NEEDS ASSESSMENT

For individuals with severe mental illness more accurate quantification of needs might contribute to the facilitation of service planning and evaluation, and promote patient recovery (Fleury et al., 2012). Various proxy measures have been developed to estimate the need for mental health services within given populations (Slade and Glover, 2001).

Epidemiological needs assessment determines the incidence and prevalence of disease in a given population. This approach does not specify the actual needs of individuals within the population but can provide an estimate of the likely numbers of individuals in need.

The proxy socio-demographic approach for the evaluation of needs is based on the determination of risk factors for a disorder in a given population. For instance, low-income, uninsured immigrants are often poverty-stricken and have a high prevalence of trauma exposure and thus are vulnerable to mental health problems. Disparities in access to mental health services highlight the importance of adapting evidence-based interventions in primary care settings that serve low income, immigrant populations (Kaltman et al., 2011). In addition, social deprivation is associated with levels of mental illness (Townsend et al., 1985; Tsang et al., 2011).

Service utilization data may be considered a proxy for need. However, current service utilization rates are an inadequate measure of local need, as they often correlate with provision - and the greater the provision, the higher the utilization rates. An additional approach, though perhaps crude, is to compare local provision with national figures.

The views of key informants (from clinicians and service planners to service users) can be gathered by individual and group interview using structured and semi-structured questionnaires, focus groups and search conferences. Lasalvia et al (2012) found that patients identified significantly fewer basic (e.g., daytime activities, food, accommodation) and functioning needs (e.g., self-care, looking after home, etc.) than staff or family members. Only fair levels of agreement were found in the three groups (average kappa was 0.48 for staff and patients, 0.54 for staff and family members, and 0.45 for patients and relatives), with patients and family members showing more areas of discrepancies in both needs and service satisfaction. The conclusion was that mental health services should routinely involve patients and their relatives when planning and evaluating psychiatric intervention and should be based on needs.

Data from the direct measurement of need among individuals can be aggregated to produce an overall estimation of need. This approach may use formal assessment instruments, such as the Camberwell Assessment of Need, Research Version (CAN-R; Slade et al., 1996).

Measurement of needs is a starting point for service planning. Needs are dynamic and must therefore be monitored over time. It is also essential to determine unmet needs and gaps in services and to link this information to service planning. Unmet health needs are often caused by barriers to health care and healthy living (Brewin, 1992, National Association of Community Health Care Centers, 2012). Mental health needs are based on poor psychological or social functioning as a consequence of mental illness. In public health and health economics, the concept of need is defined as the ability to benefit from health care (Stevens and Raftery, 1994; Asadi-Lari et al., 2005), when 'health care' is defined to include treatment, prevention, diagnosis, continuing care, rehabilitation, and palliative care. Health care outcomes also have to be considered in order to establish need. In this theoretical framework, a distinction is made between need, demand and utilization/supply. A need is the necessity for effective intervention as defined by a professional; a demand is the expression of a desire to receive treatment (or a willingness to pay for it) and utilization is the actual use or consumption of the health care provided.

Measurement of needs generally includes the following steps: (a) standardized assessment of problems in various areas or dimensions (psychopathology, functioning, basic abilities, provision of services, etc.), (b) identification of the healthcare intervention required or desired (e.g., medication, training, psychotherapy, sheltered housing, etc.), (c) identification of the support provided by family or other agencies, and finally (d) rating of the need, met or unmet, by a professional or by the patient. Because of frequent discrepancies in the assessment of needs (Wiersma, 2006), it is important to know which perspective was considered.

Studies comparing treatments actually received by patients are scant. In the European Psychiatric Services: Inputs Linked to Outcome Domains and Needs (EPSILON), multinational study the diagnosis of schizophrenia was carefully assessed in a sample of patients, using SCID (McCrone et al., 2000). Their need for care (CAN) was measured using a service receipt inventory, quality of life was measured using the Lancashire Quality of Life Profile and service satisfaction was measured with the Verona service satisfaction scale (Becker et al., 2000). Four hundred and four patients were evaluated, and they revealed wide disparities in met and unmet needs across the five participating countries, with Amsterdam and London scoring highest and Santander and Verona lowest. Satisfaction with mental health care varied across countries: it was highest in Copenhagen and lowest in London (Ruggeri et al., 2003) and was related to clinical and contextual variables.

FACTOR STRUCTURE IN THE CAMBERWELL ASSESSMENT OF NEED

To define needs for the care of people with severe mental illness, the Camberwell Assessment of Need (CAN) focuses on measuring individual and social functioning. To investigate the factor structure of the CAN, Wennstrom and colleagues (2004) used an exploratory maximum likelihood factor analysis of assessments of 741 outpatients with severe mental illness (68% had schizophrenia or another psychotic disorder). The results supported a three-factor model, comprising 13 of the 22 variables in the original CAN, with the factors corresponding to functional disability (7 variables), social loneliness (3 variables) and emotional loneliness (3 variables), while the remaining 9 variables did not load on any factor. They concluded that the three homogeneous dimensions in the CAN might represent functional disability and two aspects of social health.

THE CAMBERWELL ASSESSMENT OF NEED (RESEARCH VERSION)

Grinshpoon and associates (2008) used the CAN interview (Phelan et al., 1995) to assess patient needs. The CAN includes needs assessments in 22 domains by the patient and key caregiver. Each domain has four sections. The first section in each domain establishes whether there is a need by asking about difficulties in that particular area. The needs are rated on a three-point scale: 0=no serious problem (no need); 1=no serious or moderate problem because of continuing intervention (met need); 2=there is a current serious problem irrespective of any ongoing intervention (unmet need). The second section asks about help received from friends, relatives and other informal carers. The third section asks about how much help the person is receiving, and how much they need, from professional services. A two-point scale, 0=no and 1=yes, is used to assess whether the patient is receiving appropriate help for the problem. The term 'professional help' in the research version 2 of the CAN instrument is defined as formal help; help from relatives, friends and next-of-kin is called informal help. The instrument demonstrated high validity and inter-rater and test-retest reliability in several studies (Phelan et al., 1995; Slade et al., 1996).

Two models of the CAN were used, the 3-factor and the 5-factor models. The first includes Functional disability, Social loneliness and Emotional loneliness (Wennstrom et al., 2004) and the second includes the Basic, Social, Functioning, Health, and Service domains (Ruggeri, 1999). Functional disability includes the need domains: Looking after the home, Food, Self-care, Money, Accommodation, Transport and Telephone. This factor captures difficulties in basic functioning and in the activities of normal life. Functional disability is generally defined as any difficulty, linked to health conditions, in conducting activities of daily living (ADL) that may be subdivided into personal (excretion, washing, eating, dressing, mobility and communication), and instrumental (household activities, mobility in the wider environment and other basic activities of independent living) (McDowell and Newell, 1996).

Functional disability seems to tap both aspects of ADL: Food, Self-care and Telephone seem to be related to central aspects of personal ADL, whereas Looking after the home, Money, Accommodation and Transport are more related to aspects of instrumental ADL. These seven CAN items are also similar to central items in scales specifically designed to measure ADL (McDowell and Newell, 1996).

The other two factors, Social loneliness and Emotional loneliness, tap into two distinct aspects of social health. Social health has been defined as: "that dimension of an individual's wellbeing that concerns how he gets along with other people, how other people react to him, and how he interacts with social institutions and societal mores" (21, p.75) Thus, broadly defined, social health is associated with functioning in social roles and integration in the community, as well as with ties and close relationships on a more intimate level. One obvious sign of problems in either of these aspects of social health is loneliness. The experience of loneliness is, however, according to Weiss (1973), phenomenologically different, depending on whether it stems from social or emotional isolation. While social loneliness is a consequence of the absence of meaningful friendships, collegial relationships or links to other social networks, emotional loneliness is a result of the absence of a romantic relationship or an intimate attachment. Symptomatically, social loneliness is often associated with feelings of boredom, depression, aimlessness and marginality. Social isolation is associated not only with lower subjective wellbeing, but also with broader morbidity and mortality (Cacioppo et al., 2009). Emotional loneliness seems to be associated with apprehension, a sense of utter aloneness and a tendency to misinterpret or to exaggerate the hostile or affectionate intent of others. This typology of loneliness, first described by

Weiss (1973), has since been supported by additional studies (DiTommaso and Spinner, 1997; Russell et al., 1984; Zammuner, 2008).

In our study, in addition to the tri-dimensional model (Wennstrom et al., 2004) we also used a model of needs based on 5 aggregated problem areas in the CAN (Ruggeri et al., 2004). The conceptual domains belonging to the 5-factor model include Basic (accommodation and food), Social (company, intimate relations, sexual expression), Functioning (self-care, child care, basic education, looking after home, daytime activities, money), Health (physical health, psychological distress, psychotic symptoms, risk to self, risk to others, alcohol abuse, drug abuse), and Services (information on condition and treatment, telephone, transport, benefits).

NEEDS ASSESSMENT BY STAFF AND PATIENTS

The deinstitutionalization of people with schizophrenia and other SMI (that will be discussed in detail in Chapter 5) increases the importance of evaluating their needs (Ochoa, 2003). The importance of needs assessment for service development is widely recognized (Middelboe et al., 2001; Brunt and Hansson, 2002; Macpherson et al., 2003a,b; Ruggeri et al., 2004; Korkeila et al., 2005; Wiersma, 2006). Although there is consensus that mental health services should be provided on the basis of need (Hansson et al., 2001), the concept and measurement of needs differ greatly among professionals, patients and the patients' families.

Several studies have focused on the relationships between needs assessments by patients and staff (Ochoa et al., 2003; Macpherson et al., 2003; Foldemo et al., 2004; Korkeila et al., 2005, Lasalvia, 2012). Ochoa and colleagues (2003) chose to identify the most common needs of people with schizophrenia who live in the community, to analyze how those needs differ when evaluated by staff and by patients, to describe the kind of help patients receive, and to find out the variables that correlate with having unmet needs. Using the Camberwell Assessment of Need (CAN) to evaluate a random sample of outpatients with schizophrenia, they found that staff detected significantly more needs than patients (6.6 and 5.36, respectively). The mean number of unmet needs was also significantly higher when assessed by staff than by patients (1.82 versus 1.38). The needs most frequently detected by patients were psychotic symptoms, house upkeep, food, and information on condition and treatment. Staff most often detected needs such as psychotic symptoms, company, daytime activities, house upkeep, food, and information.

A multiple regression model found that needs had only a weak correlation with clinical variables and quality of life. The authors concluded that needs assessment complements clinical evaluation in schizophrenia.

The conceptualization and measurement of needs differ greatly not only between professionals and patients but also between the latter and their family members. Thus, Foldemo and colleagues (2004), used the CAN to assess needs of outpatients with schizophrenia, and then interviewed their parents and staff about the patient's needs. The patients scored the total severity of their needs lower than both parents and staff (a mean of 7±4 versus 9±5). Spearman's correlation for ranking individual needs as assessed by patients and parents, and patients and staff was significantly lower (0.65) than the correlation between parents and staff (0.95). Compared to the patients, the parents rated higher unmet needs involving physical health and money. The authors concluded that it is important to canvas the views of patients, parents and staff, when planning mental health care.

In Korkeila and colleagues' study (2005) the CAN structure of needs among outpatients with schizophrenia, as identified by the patients and their professional carers, was examined. The patients' quality of life, level of functioning, and psychiatric symptoms were also measured. Factor analysis identified five factors for patients and four factors for staff. A meaningful interpretation was possible in four of the five patient-related factors — skills, illness, coping, and substance abuse. The staff-related factors were skills, impairment, symptom, and substance abuse. There were significant correlations between the summary scores constructed from the factors and measures of functioning levels and symptoms. It has been concluded that the summary factor reflecting secondary needs was the most important of the identified factors among both patient and staff ratings. While in previous studies item-by-item comparisons emphasized differences between patient and staff ratings, this study also found similarities in the structures and in the correlations between the identified summary scores and measures of symptoms, functioning levels, and quality of life.

Macpherson and colleagues (2003a) used an epidemiological representative sample of patients with psychosis and an abridged version of the CAN (CANSAS) to rate staff and patient perceptions of need. The results showed that both patients and staff rated unmet needs highest in the social/relationship domains. Levels of total met and unmet needs were rated similarly by staff and patients, both as aggregate scores and by individual domain. The level of agreement between patient and staff ratings were found to be "substantial" in all domains except risk to others, where agreement was "fair" and in which staff appeared to perceive a higher risk than patients did. Staff, but not patients, rated unmet needs significantly higher in non-Caucasian groups, but no other variable correlated with unmet needs. The authors concluded that the levels of agreement between patient and staff ratings were significantly higher in their study than in earlier studies. A possible reason was that the researchers interviewed staff members who knew their patients well. Staff may have also been influenced by the awareness of how their patients perceived their needs. Joint needs assessment may thus strengthen the therapeutic alliance between patients and carers, and improve the understanding of priority needs and aid in service development. Work is needed to ensure that care is targeted explicitly towards unmet needs.

LOCAL MENTAL HEALTH SERVICES NEEDS ASSESSMENTS

Psychiatric care has moved from a hospital-oriented system to an outpatient-centered system (deinstitutionalization) and the change has underlined the importance of support alternatives. Unfortunately, service planning is rarely based on aggregated needs assessment. There is a lack of research into how population-based needs-assessment approaches can be translated into routine clinical practice.

Macpherson and colleagues (2003b) set out to investigate the level of need among those in contact with mental health services and to identify the compromises involved in the data routinely collected to inform services compared with funded research studies. They ascertained the 2-month-period prevalence of psychosis in Gloucester City. People with an ICD-10 diagnosis of functional psychosis were identified by searching general practice and mental health service records in the city. The needs of the sub-sample in contact with mental health services were assessed using the CAN. A total of 474 cases were identified, of whom 403 were in contact with mental health services. CANSAS data were collected for 225 patients, with a mean rating of 7.0 met and 3.6 unmet needs per patient. Unmet needs were higher in the non-Caucasian group. In this locality, patients with functional psychosis were largely in contact with the mental health services, were employed and were usually treated by general practitioners. A majority of the patients resided in supported accommodations. Compared to previous studies, higher levels of need were revealed. The conclusion was drawn that using research instruments to systematically assess needs in order enhance service planning is possible without major funding; however it involves compromises on established research designs.

Brunt and Hansson (2002) compared the needs for care between psychiatric inpatients and outpatients in community based sheltered housing. The CAN was administered to 75 patients and residents in different housing settings. Residents in supported-community settings had more needs for care (mean: 8.1), than patients in inpatient settings (mean: 5.8), partly because of differences in duration of illness. A greater proportion of those living in supported-community residences reported needs in the areas of psychotic symptoms, accommodation, food, daytime activities, sexual expression and caring for the home. There were no differences in numbers of unmet needs. Relatives and friends provided emotional and social support, predominantly in the areas of company and psychological distress. Living in supported-community residences, it was concluded, did not imply more unmet needs, or less adequate responses to needs from formal service systems, despite the greater number of needs reported. In some areas of need, relatives and friends play an important role in the provision of support.

CONCLUSION

Findings from the reviewed studies comparing assessments of need by staff and patients present a consistent picture (Slade et al., 1996; Slade et al., 1998; Wiersma et al., 1998; Lasalvia et al., 2000; Hansson et al., 2001; Lasalvia et al., 2012). The number of needs identified by staff and patients are broadly similar, with a tendency for staff to identify slightly more needs. However, the domains of need identified can differ substantially. There is more agreement between staff and patients when assessing domains of need with a relatively defined service response (such as accommodation) than those without (such as intimate relationships). There is more disagreement on unmet needs (domains with serious current problems irrespective of the help given) than on met needs (no or moderate problems with the help given). However, with the exception of the study by Lasalvia and colleagues (2000), the studies were conducted on outpatients.

Having argued for the active involvement of the patient in the needs assessment process and that need is a socially negotiated concept with no single 'correct' perspective (Slade, 1994, Lasalvia et al., 2012), it nonetheless remains important to examine the differences between patient and professional perspectives on need. Patients' assessments might reflect illness processes (for example, lack of insight due to psychotic illness), or social perspectives (for example, social expectation may be lower in patients living in poverty). Concern about unrealistic patient demand for limited services may result in the staff rating needs lower in order to ensure that need ratings remain within the supply potential. Differences between staff- and patient-rated needs provide potentially valuable information for care planning. For example, there is now firm evidence of the relationship between the level of collaboration in the staff-patient relationship and medication compliance (Fenton et al., 1997). An awareness of differences may also facilitate more effective service planning at the local level.

REFERENCES

Asadi-Lari M, Packham C, Gray D. Need for redefining needs. Health and quality of life outcomes. 2003;I:34. Available at: http://www.hqlo.com/content/1/1/34 (accessed on 1 January 2013).

Becker T, Knapp M, Knudsen HC, Schene AH, Tansella M, Thornicroft G, et al. Aims, outcomemeasures, study sites and patient sample. EPSILON Study 1. European Psychiatric Services: inputs linked to outcome domains and needs. *Br J Psychiatry* 2000; Suppl 39:1–7.

Brewin CR. Measuring individual needs for care and services. In: Thornicroft G, Brewin CR, Wing JK, eds. *Measuring mental health needs*. London, UK: Gaskell Royal College of Psychiatrists, 1992, pp. 220–236.

Brunt D, Hansson L. Comparison of user assessed needs for care between psychiatric inpatients and supported community residents. *Scand J Caring Sci* 2002;16:406-413.

Cacioppo JT, Fowler JH, Christakis NA. Alone in the crowd: The structure and spread of loneliness in a large social network. *J Pers Soc Psychol* 2009;97:977-991.

DiTommaso E, Spinner, B. Social and emotional loneliness: a re-examination of Weiss' typology of loneliness. *Pers Individ Dif* 1997;22:417-427.

Fenton WS, Blyler CR, Heinssen RK. Determinants of medication compliance in schizophrenia: empirical and clinical findings. *Schizophr Bull* 1997;23:637-51.

Fleury MJ, Grenier G, Bamvita JM, Tremblay J. Factors Associated with Needs of Users with Severe Mental Disorders. *Psychiatr Q* 2012 Dec 9. (Epub ahead of print).

Foldemo A, Ek AC, Bogren L. Needs in outpatients with schizophrenia, assessed by the patients themselves and their parents and staff. *Soc Psychiatry Psychiatr Epidemiol* 2004;39:381-385.

Grinshpoon A, Friger M, Orev E, Shvarts S, Kaplan Z, Abramowitz MZ, Ponizovsky AM. Relative perceptions of the needs of inpatients with schizophrenia and schizoaffective disorders. *Isr J Psychiatry Relat Sci* 2008;45:201-209.

Hansson L, Vinding HR, Mackeprang T, Sourander A, Werdelin G, Bengtsson-Tops A, Bjarnason O, Dybbro J, Nilsson L, Sandlund M, Sørgaard K, Middelboe T. Comparison of key worker and patient assessment of needs in schizophrenic patients living in the community: a Nordic multicentre study. *Acta Psychiatr Scand* 2001;103:45-51.

Kaltman S, Pauk J, Alter CL. Meeting the mental health needs of low-income immigrants in primary care: a community adaptation of an evidence-based model. *Am J Orthopsychiatry* 2011;81:543-551.

Korkeila J, Heikkila J, Hansson L, Sorgaard KW, Vahlberg T, Karlsson H. Structure of needs among persons with schizophrenia. *Soc Psychiatry Psychiatr Epidemiol* 2005;40:233-239.

Lasalvia A, Boggian I, Bonetto C, Saggioro V, Piccione G, Zanoni C, Cristofalo D, Lamonaca D. Multiple perspectives on mental health outcome: needs for care and service satisfaction assessed by staff, patients and family members. *Soc Psychiatry Psychiatr Epidemiol* 2012;47: 1035-1045.

Lasalvia A, Ruggeri M, Mazzi MA, Dall'Agnola RB. The perception of needs for care in staff and patients in community-based mental health services.The South-Verona Outcome Project 3. *Acta Psychiatr Scand* 2000;102:366-375.

Macpherson R, Varah M, Summerfield L, Foy C, Slade M. Staff and patient assessments of need in an epidemiologically representative sample of patients with psychosis--staff and patient assessments of need. *Soc Psychiatry Psychiatr Epidemiol* 2003a;38:662-667.

Macpherson R, Haynes R, Summerfield L, Foy C, Slade M. From research to practice: a local mental health services needs assessment. *Soc Psychiatry Psychiatr Epidemiol* 2003b;38:276-281.

McCrone P, Leese M, Thornicroft G, Schene A, Knudsen HC, Vazquez-Barquero JL, Tansella M, Becker T. A comparison of needs of patients with schizophrenia in five European countries: the EPSILON Study. *Acta Psychiatr Scand* 2001;103:370-379.

McDowell I & Newell C. Measuring Health. *A Guide to Rating Scales and Questionnaires* (2nd edn). Oxford: Oxford University Press, 1996.

Middelboe T, Mackeprang T, Hansson L, Werdelin G, Karlsson H, Bjarnason O, Bengtsson-Tops A, Dybbro J, Nilsson LL, Sandlund M, Sorgaard KW. The Nordic Study on schizophrenic patients living in the community. Subjective needs and perceived help. *Eur Psychiatry* 2001;16:207-214.

National Association of Community Health Care Centers . The State of Unmet Need for Primary Health Care in America, March 2012 (http://www.nachc.com/client//HealthWanted.pdf) (accessed 1.1.2013).

Ochoa S, Haro JM, Autonell J, Pendas A, Teba F, Marquez M; NEDES Group. Met and unmet needs of schizophrenia patients in a Spanish sample. *Schizophr Bull* 2003;29:201-210.

Phelan M, Slade M, Thornicroft G, Dunn G, Holloway F, Wykes T, Strathdee G, Loftus L, McCrone P, Hayward P. The Camberwell Assessment of Need: the validity and reliability of an instrument to assess the needs of people with severe mental illness. *Br J Psychiatry* 1995;167:589-595.

Ruggeri M, Lasalvia A, Bisoffi G, Thornicroft G, Vazquez-Barquero JL, Becker T, et al. Satisfaction with mental health services among people with schizophrenia in five European sites: results from the EPSILON Study. *Schizophr Bull* 2003;29:229–245.

Ruggeri M, Leese M, Slade M, Bonizzato P, fontecedro L, Tansella M. demographic clinical social and service variables associated with higher needs for care in community psychiatric service patients. The South Verona Outcome Project 8. *Soc Psychiatry Psychiatr Epidemiol* 2004; 39:60-68.

Ruggeri M. (Camberwell assessment of need (CAN). Preliminary introduction). *Epidemiol Psichiatr Soc.* 1999;8(2):131-167. (Italian).

Russell D, Cutrona CE, Rose J, et al. Social and emotional loneliness: an examination of Weiss's typology of loneliness. *J Pers Soc Psychol* 1984;46:1313-1321.

Russell R. Social health: An attempt to clarify this dimension of well-being. *Int J Health Educ* 1973;16:74–82.

Slade M, Glover G. The needs of the people with mental disorders. In *Textbook of Community Psychiatry*, Graham Thornicroft, George Szmukler (eds), Oxford: Oxford University Press, 2001.

Slade M, Phelan M, Thornicroft G, Parkman S. The Camberwell Assessment of Need (CAN): Comparison of assessments by staff and patients of the needs of the severely mentally ill. *Soc Psychiatry Psychiatr Epidemiol* 1996;31:109–113.

Slade M, Phelan M, Thornicroft G. A comparison of needs assessed by staff and by an epidemiologically representative sample of patients with psychosis. *Psychol Med* 1998;28:543–550.

Slade M. Needs assessment. Involvement of staff and users will help to meet needs. *Br J Psychiatry* 1994;165:293-296.

Stevens A, Raftery J. Health care needs assessment. *The epidemiologically based needs assessment reviews*. Oxford and New York: Radcliffe Medical Press, 1994, pp. 11–30.

Townsend P, Simpson D, Tibbs N. Inequalities in health in the city of Bristol: a preliminary review of statistical evidence. *Int J Health Serv* 1985;15:637-663.

Tsang HW, Li D, Tsui MC, Chung RC, Wong AH, Li SM, Fung KM, Yiu MG. The Perceived Rehabilitation Needs of People with Schizophrenia in Hong Kong: Perspectives from Consumers and Care-givers. Adm *Policy Ment Health* 2011 Dec 13. (Epub ahead of print).

Weiss R. *The experience of emotional and social isolation.* Cambridge (MA): MIT press, 1973.

Wennstrom E, Sorbom D, Wiesel FA. Factor structure in the Camberwell Assessment of Need. *Br J Psychiatry* 2004;185:505-510.

Wiersma D, Nienhuis FJ, Giel R, Slooff CJ. Stability and change in needs of patients with schizophrenic disorders: a 15- and 17-year follow-up from first onset of psychosis, and a comparison between 'objective' and 'subjective' assessments of needs for care. *Soc Psychiatry Psychiatr Epidemiol* 1998;33:49-56.

Wiersma D. Needs of people with severe mental illness. *Acta Psychiatr Scand* 2006;113 (Suppl. 429):115–119.

Zammuner VL. Italians' Social and Emotional Loneliness: The Results of Five Studies. *Int J Human Soc Sci* 2008;3:108-120.

Chapter 3

MATCHING NEEDS WITH MENTAL HEALTH SERVICES

ABSTRACT

In this chapter the need profile of a homogeneous group of schizophrenia patients who were hospitalized for the treatment of severe mental illness is presented. The needs of these patients were comprehensively assessed in relation to selected sociodemographic and clinical characteristics as well as to measures of their psychopathological symptoms, functioning, general wellbeing and life satisfaction. As previously mentioned, mental health services should be provided on the basis of psychiatric patients' needs. By delineating the discrepancies in need assessments and focusing on patient perceived needs, appropriate service delivery of those needs will be introduced. Chapter four will familiarize the reader with psychiatric services existing in Israel in order to meet these needs.

DIVERSITY OF MENTAL HEALTH SERVICES

Aside from pharmacological research reports, recent literature on the care of patients with severe mental disorders has focused on evidence-based practices that include assertive community treatment (ACT), cognitive behavior therapy (CBT) for psychosis, cognitive remediation, family psycho-education, illness self-management training, social skills training, and supported employment (Mueser et al., 2013). Additional promising practices include healthy lifestyle interventions, cognition training, supported education, supported housing, family therapy (Pharoah et al., 2010), cognitive behavior therapy (Pilling et al., 2002), and assertive outreach (Billings et al., 2003; Fakhoury et al., 2007).The efficacy of deinstitutionalization in small units (Grinshpoon et al., 2003, 2006; Nordentoft et al., 2010) has also been widely discussed.

Bustillo et al (2001) concluded that:

"Relatively simple, long-term psycho-educational family therapy should be available to the majority of persons suffering from schizophrenia. Assertive community training programs ought to be offered to patients with frequent relapses and hospitalizations, especially if they have limited family support. Patients with schizophrenia can clearly improve their social competence with social skills training, which may translate into a more adaptive functioning in the community. For patients interested in working, rapid placement with ongoing support offers the best opportunity for maintaining a regular job in the community. Cognitive behavior therapy may benefit the large number of patients who continue to experience disabling psychotic symptoms despite optimal pharmacological treatment" (page 163).

Compared with those receiving medication only, patients with early-stage schizophrenia who receive medication together with psychosocial intervention have a lower rate of treatment discontinuation or change, a lower risk of relapse, and improved insight, quality of life, and social functioning (Guo et al., 2010).

UNIVERSAL AND SPECIFIC NEEDS OF PEOPLE WITH MENTAL DISORDERS

Although people with mental health problems have some specific needs, the majority of their needs are similar to those of people without mental illness. As previously mentioned, needs assessment should be both an integral part of clinical practice and a component of service evaluation.

The WHO's Illness, Disability and Handicap (IDH) classification of consequences of disease and injury has been used to classify mental health needs on three levels. Primary needs are associated with psychopathology or impairment. Secondary needs arise from disabilities and restrictions on personal activities that may be directly caused by the impairment. Tertiary needs concern the social consequences of illness, the handicaps that affect one's interactions with his surroundings (WHO, 1980). Psychiatric disorders are associated with a wide range of needs in the social and personal domains that are not necessarily considered within the realm of 'the need for care', however these domains are highly pertinent for people living with mental disorders (Wing et al., 2001).

Need is a subjective concept and there are often different but equally valid perceptions about the presence or absence of a specific need. It is very important, therefore, to identify the differences in perception of need between mental health service users and their professional care-givers (Lasalvia et al., 2000; Grinshpoon et al., 2008). Once differences are identified, negotiations between providers and users can progress toward a care plan. Once the intervention has been devised an agent can be chosen to provide the setting in which user and care-giver can interact (Mangen and Brewin, 1991).

The distinction must be preserved between need (the ability to benefit in some way from health care), demand (wishes expressed by the service user), and the provision and utilization of services (Stevens and Gabbay, 1991). These will never be perfectly matched but mismatch can be minimized as long as service development adheres to two fundamental principles:

- Local services should be shaped by the specific needs of the population rather than provided in line with a national template or historical pattern.
- Sufficient resources should be provided for effective interventions.

NEEDS AND DEMOGRAPHIC, CLINICAL, SOCIAL AND SERVICE PROFILES

Middelboe and colleagues (2001) used the Camberwell Assessment of Need to measure subjective needs and perceived help in a community sample of persons diagnosed with schizophrenia. The mean number of reported needs was 6.2 and the mean number of unmet needs, 2.6. The prevalence of needs varied substantially between need areas from 3.6% (telephone) to 84.0% (psychotic symptoms). The rate of satisfaction, estimated as the percentage of persons satisfied with the help provided in a given area of need, ranged from 20.0% (telephone) to 80.6% (food). Unmet needs as a proportion of total needs was highest in need areas pertaining to social and interpersonal functioning. In a majority of need areas the patients received more help from formal services than from relatives, but in the areas of social relations the informal network provided substantial help. In general, the patients reported a need for help from services which significantly exceeded the actual amount of help received. In a linear regression model, symptom load as assessed with the Brief Psychiatric Rating Scale (BPRS; Overall and Gorham, 1962) and impaired functioning as assessed with the Global Assessment of Functioning (GAF; American Psychiatric Association, 2000) were significant predictors of need status, explaining 30% of the variance in total needs and 20% of the variance in unmet needs. It was concluded that the mental health system failed to detect and alleviate needs in several areas of major importance to schizophrenia patients. Therefore, enhanced collaboration between the formal care system and the informal network is necessary in order to systematically map patients' need profiles and minimize the gap between perceived needs and received help.

Ruggeri and colleagues (2004) investigated a representative sample of patients attending a community-based psychiatric service in order to identify the needs profiles of patients with higher levels of care needs. Their approach was based on calculating the correlations between a full range of demographic, clinical, social and service variables. The sample included 268 patients using mental health services in South Verona, Italy. Cross-sectional assessments of needs (using the CAN), symptoms, disability, functioning, quality of life, service use and satisfaction with care were made and analyzed by linear regression. A model that included 'being male', 'being unemployed', 'having high levels of symptoms and disability', 'having low functioning and self-reported quality of life', and 'having a high number of outpatient and community contacts' accounted for 67% of the variance in the total level of need. It was concluded that patients who meet any of these criteria would be more likely to have higher needs, a conclusion which has implications for clinical practice and audit. The authors also concluded that the CAN is a good overall measure of the number and the severity of a patient's problems in several key areas of everyday life.

NEEDS AND SYMPTOM DIMENSIONS IN SCHIZOPHRENIA

Severity of symptoms is one of the most consistent factors associated with the number of patient needs. Several studies have found that outpatients with schizophrenia with more severe symptoms had a greater number of total and unmet needs (Alvarado et al., 2012; McCrone et al., 2001; Foldemo and

Borgen, 2002; Middelboe et al., 2001). Ochoa et al (2005) analyzed the association between symptom dimensions in schizophrenia and number and type of met and unmet needs. A sample of 231 outpatients randomly selected from a register that included all patients treated in five mental health care centers (MHCC) was evaluated by the CAN questionnaire and the PANSS. They found that the number of needs correlated to overall severity of psychopathology, i.e., patients with more symptoms had significantly more total needs and unmet needs, as well. A multiple linear regression model showed that the disorganized and excited dimensions of the PANSS were the most important components for explaining the variance in number of needs. Type of need was related to subtypes of schizophrenia, and especially with disorganized and excited symptoms.

MENTAL HEALTH NEEDS AND QUALITY OF LIFE

Few studies have investigated the relationship between care needs and subjective quality of life among patients with schizophrenia (Hansson et al., 2003; Slade et al., 2005, Lasalvia et al., 2005). Hansson and colleagues (2003) examined this relationship in a cross-sectional multi-center study of patients diagnosed with schizophrenia from 10 centers in Nordic countries. Needs in 22 domains were investigated by interviews with key workers and their patients, using the CAN scale, and appraising quality of life by the Lancashire Quality of Life Profile. The results showed that key workers rated needs slightly higher than patients. A higher level of unmet need, as rated by both key workers and patients, correlated with a poorer overall subjective quality of life, whereas met needs showed no such association. A regression analysis, controlling for the patients' clinical and social characteristics, also showed that higher unmet needs were associated with a worse quality of life. Regression analyses of the relationship of unmet needs in specific life domains and overall quality of life showed that patient-rated unmet needs in five domains accounted for 17% of the explained variance in overall quality of life. More than half of this variance was related to unmet needs in the domain of social relationships. Hence, unmet needs are of specific importance in needs assessment and that particular attention must be paid to seeking solutions for unmet needs when planning interventions and services in order to facilitate improvement in quality of life. In this context, specific attention should also be paid to unmet needs in the domains of social relationships and appropriate living accommodations.

In a longitudinal study, Slade and colleagues (2005) tested the hypotheses (a) that higher patient-rated unmet needs is associated with lower individual quality of life assessments by patients over time, and (b) that a reduction in patient-rated unmet needs precipitates improvement in quality of life. A total of 101 individuals using adult mental health services were asked to complete 6-monthly questionnaires, including quality of life (MANSA) and unmet need (abridged CAN) assessments. Seventy-three patients provided 240 pairs of consecutive assessments. Random effects regression models indicated an impact on current quality of life for both average levels of unmet needs and changes in unmet needs over the past month. The authors concluded that changes in patient-rated unmet needs may lead to changes in quality of life.

Lasalvia and colleagues (2005) used a four-year prospective longitudinal design on a cohort of patients from the South Verona Community-based Mental Health Service in order to investigate the impact of meeting needs for care (as assessed by both patients and mental health professionals) on subjective quality of life. Needs were assessed by the CAN (both staff and patient versions) and subjective quality of life was measured by the Lancashire Quality of Life Profile. The study revealed that improvement in patients' clinical conditions, together with reduction in patient-rated unmet needs in the social domain, predicted an increase in subjective quality of life over the four-year period, whereas changes in staff-rated needs did not show any association with change in subjective quality of life. Thus, meeting self-perceived social needs has a more important role in ensuring a better quality of life for people with mental disorders than just symptom reduction. A policy of actively and adequately addressing patient-rated needs should be implemented in order to improve client quality of life.

Recently, Ritsner and Grinshpoon (2013) examined the relationship between unmet needs and quality of life (QOL) across time, of patients with schizophrenia (SZ) and schizoaffective (SA) disorder. They evaluated ninety-five stable SZ/SA patients using the Quality of Life Enjoyment and Life Satisfaction Questionnaire, the Positive and Negative Syndromes Scale (PANSS), the Multidimensional Scale of Perceived Social Support (MSPSS), and the Coping Inventory for Stressful Situations (CISS). Study participants were followed for a decade, and at the ten year evaluation, patients completed the Camberwell Assessment of Need Scale. Correlation and multivariate regression analyses revealed that the number of unmet needs negatively correlated with Q-LES-Q domains, however their predictive value for general quality of life did not reach significant levels controlling for MSPSS, and CISS scores. Individual needs included assistance with psychological distress, daytime activities, welfare benefits, physical health, food and intimate relationships, which emerged as a significant predictor of current general QOL, even after controlling for PANSS, MSPSS, and CISS scores. Patients whose conditions had deteriorated and were dissatisfied with their general QOL over time expressed many more unmet needs compared to those who were satisfied and reported improved QOL. Individual unmet needs concerning daytime activities, psychological distress, psychotic symptoms, information about treatment, company, and money were associated with reduced and unsatisfactory general QOL. The authors concluded that unmet needs of SZ/SA patients strongly correlate with quality of life outcome across time, and the pattern of individual unmet needs rather than the number of unmet needs has a greater predictive value for current subjective quality of life. Hence, considering that one of the main goals of mental health care is to improve psychiatric patients' quality of life, actively addressing patient-rated needs is crucial.

THE PATIENT NEEDS PROFILE

In a series of studies that investigated the relationship between perceived patient needs, clinical symptoms and service-provision, we described the need profile of a homogeneous group of schizophrenia inpatients, and comprehensively assessed the needs of these patients in relation to selected sociodemographic and clinical characteristics and measures of their psychopathological symptoms, functioning, general wellbeing and life satisfaction. Results of these studies have been published in the scientific literature and are cited below (Grinshpoon and Ponizovsky 2008; Grinshpoon et al., 2008).

The studies were performed in Beersheba Mental Health Center, a government hospital affiliated to Ben-Gurion University of the Negev. Participants were 52 consecutively-admitted voluntary inpatients age 18-65, admitted from the community who met ICD-10 criteria for the diagnosis of schizophrenia (F 20) or schizoaffective disorders (F 25) and were able to provide written informed consent for participation in the study. Exclusion criteria were acute psychotic state at admission or coexisting mental retardation, dementia or other severe organic brain pathology. The sociodemographic profile of the sample was as follows: 65.4% male, mean age 38.1 years (SD=10.8 years, range=21-62 years), 92% Jewish; 61%Israel-born; 62% single, 23% divorced, 15% married; 94% had secondary school education, 40% competed high school; 31% were employed. The clinical profile of the sample was as follows: of the 52 patients, 26 met ICD-10 criteria for schizophrenia and 26 for schizoaffective disorders. Mean age at onset of the illness, defined as age at first psychiatric admission, was 25 years (SD=10). The mean duration of illness was 166 months (SD=117). At data collection all patients were hospitalized, mean length of the current hospitalization was 22.2 days (SD=20), and the mean total number of psychiatric admissions was 14 (SD=12). For the entire sample, the PANSS mean total score was 77.3 (SD=19.3); the Positive Scale score was 19.9 (SD=6.7), the Negative Scale score was 18.6 (SD=6.8), and the General Psychopathology scale score was 39.4 (SD=9.4). In addition, the General Life Functioning mean total score was 54.3 (SD=10.5) and the General Health Questionnaire mean score was 39.3 (SD=4.4).

The proportion of patients that reported a need within a CAN domain ranged from 1.9% (Telephone) to 73.1% (Information on condition and treatment). Unmet needs were particularly prevalent in the domains Information on condition and treatment (48.1% of the full sample), Benefits (36.5%), Sexual expression (26.9%), Company, Intimate relationships, and Psychological distress (each 25%), and Psychotic symptoms (23.1%).

The ratio of unmet to total needs was calculated in order to examine for neglected need domains or where intervention was unsuccessful. Unmet need predominated in the need domains of Transport (100%), Benefits (90.5%), Safety to others (80%), Sexual expression (73.7%), and Daytime activities (71.4%).

Research studies using the CAN generate on average 5–8 needs with the lowest ratio of met to unmet needs 2:1 (Phelan et al., 1995; Arvidsson, 2003; Hansson et al., 1995; Issakidis and Teesson, 1999; Leese et al., 1998; Mccrone et al., 2001; Slade et al., 1998; Slade et al., 1999; Wiersma and Van Busschbach, 2001; Zahid and Ohaeri, 2013). The numbers are higher among hospitalized patients, patients suffering from schizophrenia and those living in urbanized areas. Patterns of need may be explained in part by service provision, e.g., sheltered accommodations in comparison to a day center with activities. Unmet needs also frequently relate to the domains of Psychotic symptoms, Company, Daytime activities and Psychological distress.

The ratio of unmet to total needs, i.e., the more congruent the network with patient needs, the lower the proportion of unmet needs, is an indicator of the degree to which professional and private networks match the patient's need profile.

Frequency of unmet needs is a particularly critical indicator. As stated in the CAN manual (Slade et al., 1999), serious unmet needs reported by patients pose a major challenge to the health care system.

In our study (Grinshpoon et al., 2008) more than 25% of patients reported unmet needs in the domains of information on condition and treatment, benefits, sexual expression, intimate relationships, company, and psychological distress. The domains of social and interpersonal relations show higher unmet needs, suggesting that there is ineffective service provision in these domains. Patients indicated that in these particular need areas help was more forthcoming from informal sources of social support (relatives/friends) than from formal services and indicated that relatives and friends play a more significant supportive role in these particular domains than hospital staff

The high rate of dissatisfaction with the help provided by services within the need domain of Physical health is indicative of the well-established fact of increased physical morbidity among persons with mental disorders (Scott et al., 2012; Briskman et al., 2012; Druss and von Esenwein, 2006). In particular, patients with schizophrenia are at higher risk for medical illnesses than people in the general population (Davidson, 2002) and more than half of patients with schizophrenia have comorbid chronic medical illness (Felker et al., 1996; Chwastiak et al., 2006). The increased risk of cardiovascular diseases and sudden death among people with schizophrenia highlights a need for preventive services, which is further underscored by the numerous system- and patient-related barriers to preventive treatment. Clinicians must not only be aware that the risk factors are modifiable but must also, in conjunction with other health care specialists, learn to manage the obstacles to prevention (Goff et al., 2005; Briskman et al., 2012; Levinson et al., 2008). According to the current reform in psychiatric services in Israel, family doctors have become the key figures in the treatment of mentally ill patients. This innovation allows for better monitoring of physical health, diagnosis and comprehensive care.

Given the increasing emphasis on psychoeducation as a means for improving outcome in schizophrenia (Merinder, 2000; Xia et al., 2011), the finding that the most prevalent unmet need is for information on condition and treatment (48%), despite the help received from formal and informal sources of support, shows that focused intervention is necessary. Also, the high prevalence of the needs for sexual expression and intimate relations are indicative of dysfunctions in this domain and has obvious consequences on their quality of life (McCann Aggregated analysis showed that basic needs were met for most patients (70%), while most unmet needs were concentrated in the areas of Health (87%), Services (83%) and Social (75%) and Functioning (65%) domains.

The findings that basic needs were satisfied for most patients should be considered in the context of deinstitutionalization, an unprecedented process of transition from care in traditional mental health hospitals to care in community-based facilities. The ideology behind deinstitutionalization was that long-stay inpatients could be discharged if adequate community facilities were available, thus leading to a steep decline in the need for inpatient beds (Holloway et al., 1996; Clifford et al., 1991; Lelliott and Wing 1994). However, in many countries psychiatric hospital beds were dramatically reduced before community based facilities were adequately developed. As a result, many former psychiatric inpatients found themselves in the community, homeless and socially deprived (Lehman et al., 1999; Hamden et al., 2011; Woollcott, 2008), and 'new long-stay' patients accumulated in psychiatric hospitals, accumulating long hospitalization duration through recurrent hospital stays (Donnelly et al., 1997; Franz et al., 2010; Shepherd, 1998; Thornicroft et al., 1992).

In Israel, the mental health reform was implemented relatively late. Although the process of deinstitutionalization began as early as the early 1980's, the Rehabilitation Act that provides a basket of rehabilitation services for individuals with mental disorders came into effect only in the year 2000. Having learned from the negative experiences of other countries, Israel attempted to build an adequate supportive mental health infrastructure in the community prior to the significant reduction in the number of inpatient beds (from 1.17 per 1000 population in 1996 to 0.45 in 2006 – Central Bureau of Statistics, 2004). In parallel with the reduction in the number of psychiatric beds, the number of hostels and sheltered homes has rapidly increased: in 1996 there were 17 hostels and 1050 people in sheltered housing settings in the country. By 2005 these figures had reached 110 and 5,300, respectively (National Psychiatric Hospitalization Registry). This rehabilitation-oriented policy has thus provided residential care to more than 5,300 chronic psychiatric patients (of course, not all of them had been in long-term inpatient care), 70% of them were diagnosed schizophrenia (Grinshpoon et al., 2003). The Rehabilitation Act, 2000, has had a beneficial effect on the opportunities of long-stay psychiatric patients to resettle in the community (Grinshpoon et al., 2006).

THE HELP RECEIVED

The percentage of patients that received 'some' or 'much' help from services ranged from 1.9% (Sexual expression, Intimate relationships, Alcohol, Looking after the home, and Accommodation) to 26.9% (Information on condition and treatment). The corresponding figures for help received from relatives and/or friends ranged from 7.7% (Daytime activities, Sexual expression, Childcare, Basic education, and Transport) to 32.7% (Information on condition and treatment) (Grinshpoon et al., 2008).

The number of patients that received services was lower than the number of patients in need of services. This was particularly true for the domains of health, that were characterized with a high number of unmet needs: Physical health (3 of 9), Psychological distress (8 of 20), Psychotic symptoms (9 of 15), Information on condition and treatment (14 of 23), Safety to self (7 of 12), and Safety to others (4 of 7). To an even greater extent, was it the case for needs in the domain of interpersonal relationships: Company (7 of 13), Intimate relationships (1 of 9), and Sexual expression (1 of 10). Interestingly, the help received from relatives and/or friends was higher in the same need domains, i.e., Physical health and Interpersonal relationships. However, relative to other need domains, more patients in these domains responded that they received the right type of help and were more satisfied with the help obtained (Grinshpoon et al., 2008).

AGGREGATED NEED AREAS

To make it easier to draw comparisons between patients', staffers', and relatives' perceptions of needs, following Lasalvia and colleagues' study (2005), we grouped the CAN 22 need items into 5 aggregated areas: Basic, Social, Functioning, Health, and Service needs. Most commonly a patient's needs concentrated in a single area. In the Health need area only 14% of patients had no problems, however 86% of the patients had from 1 to 7 unmet needs and 58% had as many as 3-7 unmet needs. Similarly in the Service need area only 17% of patients had no complaints, while 83% had from 1 to 4 unmet needs. In contrast, in the Basic need area as many as 69% of patients had no complaints, whereas 31% had one and two unmet needs. The most frequent combinations of need areas were Health and Service (15%) and Health, Social and Functioning (8%). Thus, although the basic needs of most patients are generally met, social, health, and service needs are not (Grinshpoon et al., 2008).

DIFFERENT PERCEPTIONS OF PATIENTS' NEEDS

To test the hypothesis that staff and family members would assess patients' unmet needs higher than the patients themselves, we compared the number of patients' needs, as rated by the patients, by a psychiatric ward nurse and by the patients' relatives and/or friends. The null hypothesis that there would be no difference in assessments of unmet needs by the patients, staff and relatives was confirmed for 16 of the 22 CAN need domains. Assessment of unmet needs differed significantly between patients and staff members in the remaining six domains. . The patients rated total needs higher than the staff in only two domains (Information on condition and treatment and Benefits; p=.014 and p<.001, respectively), The staff rated need for Intimate relationships (p=.032), Safety to others (p<.005), Self-care (p=.017), and Daytime activities (p<.0001) higher than the patients (Grinshpoon et al., 2008) Patients reported significantly fewer needs in the domains of Safety to self (p=.025) and Psychotic symptoms (p=.003) as well as Benefits (p<.01), Daytime activities (p<.0001), Safety to others (p=.017) and Self-care (p<.0001) (Grinshpoon et al., 2008).

The concept of need assumes a degree of subjectivity and there is need for care or support in situations involving reduced physical, psychological or social functioning. Furthermore, if need is viewed as a subjective concept, the identification and assessment of severity of need may be influenced by the perspective of the assessor. Assessment of needs by psychiatric nurses and their patients may differ for various reasons. Patients and professionals have different priorities and different sources of information for defining needs (Landis and Koch, 1977). Studies that evaluated multiple perspectives concerning needs as assessed by staff, patients and families have revealed discrepancies between staff and patients. Lasalvia et al (2012) found that patients identified significantly fewer basic (e.g., daytime activities, food, accommodation) and functioning needs (e.g., self-care, looking after home, etc.) than staff or family members. Only fair levels of agreement were found in the three groups (average kappa was 0.48 for staff and patients, 0.54 for staff and family members, and 0.45 for patients and relatives), with patients and family members showing more areas of discrepancies in both needs and service satisfaction.

Slade et al (1996; 1998) found that patients and staff reported a similar number of needs but in different life domains and patients identified a wider range of needs (Slade et al., 1998). Disparities concerning the number and type of needs reported by patients, case managers, and families are statistically significant but inconclusive (Wiersma, 2006).

In line with previous studies (Macpherson et al., 2003; Slade et al., 1996), we did not find significant differences between the perceptions of patients and staff members on most need domains. Substantial discrepancies occurred in only 6 of 22 CAN domains. The patients rated the needs for Information on condition, treatment and Benefits higher than the staff, and the staff rated the patients' needs for Intimate relationships, Safety to others, Self-care, and Daytime activities domains higher that the patients. Analogous differences occurred between the patients and their relatives or friends in the same need areas.

Higher estimation of the needs for Self-care and Daytime activities by staff members could be explained by a paternalist approach to patients with severe mental illness, which still persists in many psychiatric hospitals, and implies that the staff can best identify the patients' needs. The findings of this study call for replacing the paternalist attitude with a partnership approach.

The results concerning Safety to others are consistent with Macpherson and colleagues' data (2000) and imply a higher perception of risk to others among staff than among patients.

When needs assessments in aggregated need areas were compared among patients, staff and relatives, patients reported significantly less unmet needs in the Social loneliness domain than both staff and relatives/friends, but not in the Emotional loneliness domain, where all the raters' assessments were similar. Similarly, patients rated their needs lower in the Functioning and Health areas than both staff and relatives. The results of this aggregated needs analysis confirm findings that patients are prone to underrate social, health and functioning problems caused by their mental illness. Alternatively, staff and relatives may be prone to overemphasize patients' disabilities. To test which view is more accurate, we performed a correlation analysis, that revealed that although there was a significant negative correlation between CAN and Global Life Functioning total scores ($r=-.31$), the dimensional scores on both instruments showed no correlation.

We repeated the analysis using the CAN 3-factor and 5-factor models and analysis of variance (one-way ANOVA), with post-hoc single comparisons by paired t-tests. ANOVA results were significant for the dimensions of Functional disability ($p<0.05$) and Social loneliness ($p<0.05$) in the CAN 3-

factor model, and for the areas of Functioning (p<0.01) and Health (p<0.001) in the CAN 5-factor model.

The ANOVA result was marginally significant for the Service need area (p=0.06). Post-hoc single comparisons showed that all differences between the patients, staffers and relatives in the perception of the patient's needs went in the same direction: the patients reported less unmet needs than staffers and relatives did.

NEEDS BY DEMOGRAPHIC AND CLINICAL VARIABLES

Association between the total mean number of unmet needs in all 22 domains of the CAN and the sociodemographic and clinical characteristics of the patients were studied (Grinshpoon and Ponizovsky, 2008). There were no significant differences in the mean number of unmet needs between male and female patients (p=0.15), age groups (p=0.33), marital status (p=0.88), schooling levels (p=0.16) and immigrant status (p=0.45). The only significant difference was found for employment status, where the number of unmet needs among the unemployed was twice higher than that among employed patients (p=0.015).

There were no significant differences in the number of unmet needs between patients diagnosed with schizophrenia and schizoaffective disorders (p=0.48). Likewise, the number of unmet needs did not vary significantly by age at first admission (p=0.51). No significant correlation was found between the number of unmet needs and duration of the illness (r=-0.26), total number of psychiatric admissions (r=-0.26), and length of current hospital stay (r=0.26; all p>0.05).

Ruggeri and colleagues (2004) examined the needs profile of community psychiatric service patients with higher care needs by analyzing the correlations between needs and demographic, clinical and social variables. They found that, of the demographic variables, only male gender and unemployed status were associated with the needs profile. Gender, but not age or age at onset of disorder, was an important determinant of patient needs. Women presented less needs than men, a finding attributable to their better social functioning (Usall et al., 2002; Leung and Chue, 2000) but not to differences in the severity of symptoms, since the researchers did not find gender differences in symptomatology (Usall et al., 2002). Recently, however, Meesters et al (2013) revealed that, the needs of elderly patients were similar to those of younger patients. One hundred and fourteen individuals with schizophrenia spectrum disorders (mean age 69 years) reported an average of 7.6 needs, of which 6.1 were met and 1.5 were unmet. Staff members reported slightly more met and unmet needs. Patients and staff showed consensus on the presence of most needs, but discrepancies existed in individual need areas. Psychological and social needs were more frequently unmet than environmental and physical needs. The number of unmet needs correlated with several patient variables, with the strongest association found for self-reported quality of life. These results differ from earlier reported findings by Middelboe and colleagues (2001) that indicated that age is related to both severity of symptoms and needs, and from Hansson and colleagues' data (1995) which also suggested that older individuals have more needs.

Grinshpoon and Ponizovsky (2008) found that almost all the socio-demographic characteristics studied, such as ethnicity, schooling, marital and immigrant status, did not correlate with the number of unmet needs. However, consistent with Ruggeri and colleagues' findings, we also found that unemployed patients had twice the total number of unmet needs of their employed counterparts. This finding has important implications for mental health policy, as it shows a need to replace conventional rehabilitation strategies using sheltered employment by finding patients employment in competitive jobs. In recent years, the Israel Ministry of Health has invested substantial effort in developing differentiated rehabilitation programs, which, in accordance with patients' wishes and capacity, will prepare them for either supported or competitive employment.

NEEDS BY CLINICAL SYMPTOMS AND FUNCTIONING

In order to define the needs for services, the CAN focuses on measuring personal and social functioning. A model of the CAN developed by Wennstrom and associates (2004) was used to examine the relationships between needs, clinical symptoms and other measures of disability. Recall that this model includes three factors: functional disability, social loneliness and emotional loneliness. The functional disability dimension captures difficulties in basic functions and activities in normal living and consists of 7 need items, such as Looking after the home, Food, Self-care, Money, Accommodation, Transport, and Telephone. The other two factors, Social loneliness and Emotional loneliness, tap into two distinct aspects of social health. The former is made up of Company, Daytime activities and Psychological distress, while the latter consists of Sexual expression, Intimate relationships and Safety to others.

Clinical symptoms were measured using two PANSS-based model of psychopathology: the 3-factor and 5-factor models. The former is a traditional model consisting of positive symptom dimension, negative symptom dimension, and general psychopathological symptoms. The latter includes in addition to positive and negative symptom dimensions, disorganized, affective and excited dimensions. Finally, the Global Life Functioning inventory comprises two dimensions: general wellbeing and functioning scales.

To test the hypothesis that unmet needs would be higher among those with higher levels of distress and also among those with lower levels of wellbeing, functioning and quality of life, Spearman's rank correlation coefficients between the CAN dimension scores and the GLF and PANSS symptom dimensions scores were calculated. A few significant positive correlations of modest magnitude were found. The CAN total score was significantly and negatively correlated with the GLF total score ($r= -.31$) and positively with the GHQ-12 total score ($r= .41$) and the PANSS negative and general symptom scales (both $r= .30$). Likewise, the CAN functional disability factor correlated significantly and positively with PANSS negative symptom dimensions ($r= .49$) and general symptom dimensions ($r= .39$), and total score ($r= .37$) (Grishpoon and Ponizovsky, 2008).

To test the hypothesis that unmet needs would be higher among those with higher levels of psychopathological symptoms, we used the CAN as a categorical dichotomized variable indicating the presence/absence of unmet need. Of all 22 need domains, significant differences between PANSS dimension scores were found only in nine items, with higher PANSS scores occurring among those who had higher unmet needs. More severe affective symptoms were noted among patients with unmet needs in the following domains: Accommodation ($p<.05$), Physical health ($p<.05$), Information on condition and treatment ($p<.05$), Alcohol ($p<.05$), Drugs ($p<.05$), Money ($p<.05$), and Benefits ($p<.01$). In addition, higher levels of negative symptoms were found in patients who had unmet needs in the domains of Information on condition and treatment ($p<.05$) and Transport ($p<.05$). More severe disorganized symptoms were found in those with unmet needs in the domains of Physical health ($p<.05$), Basic education ($p<.01$) and Transport ($p<.05$), and excited symptoms in those with problems in Information on condition and treatment ($p<.05$) and Money ($p<.05$). Interestingly, no significant differences were found in positive symptom scores among those with presence /absence of needs in any CAN domain.

We found that selected clinical features, such as ICD-10 diagnosis (schizophrenia/schizoaffective disorder), age at first admission, overall duration of illness, lifetime number of psychiatric admissions and length of current hospital stay were not associated with the number of unmet needs. As these variables are indicators of the long-term course of an illness, these findings do not demonstrate a relationship between unmet needs and the course of illness.

By contrast, as expected, an important relationship between the presence of psychiatric and psychosocial needs and severity of psychopathology was revealed. In line with other authors (McCrone et al., 2001; Middelboe et al., 2001), with the patients in this study that had higher severity of overall psychopathology had more needs and especially more unmet needs. More specifically, CAN Functional disability dimension scores were significantly correlated to PANSS Negative symptom and General psychopathology scale scores.

As previously reported (Grinshpoon and Ponizovsky, 2008), using the 5-dimensional model of psychopathology, we found that a higher need profile was related to a greater severity of the PANSS affective, disorganized, negative and excited symptom dimensions. It was noteworthy, however, that no relationship was found between any CAN domain and the PANSS Positive symptom dimension. The findings are consistent with other studies that have shown that BPRS items covering anxiety, depressive and negative symptoms are associated with higher needs in most CAN domains, while the items covering positive symptoms are associated only with some specific need domain (Ruggeri et al., 2004). However, our findings gave only partial support to studies that concluded that disorganized and excited PANSS dimensions are more important in predicting the presence of unmet needs than positive, negative and affective symptoms (Ochoa et al., 2005).

Relevant relationships were found between symptom dimensions and need domains. First, the relationship between affective (depressive) symptoms and serious problems in the domains of physical health, alcohol and drug abuse seems easy to explain by the association of depression with somatization disorder (Greed and Barsky, 2004; Teesson et al., 2011) and/or attempts at self-treatment for depressive mood with psychoactive substances (Hendrickson et al., 2004; Majumder et al., 2012). It is difficult to explain the relation between affective symptoms and the needs for Accommodation, Benefits, Money and Information on condition and treatment. One possible explanation could be the substantial cognitive distortions of perception caused by depressive symptoms in schizophrenia (Rector and Beck, 2002). It was surprising however, that no relationship was found between affective (depressive) symptoms and Safety to self since depression is a very well known risk factor for suicide and self-injury. Despite this lack, the assessment of affective symptoms should also be present in the evaluation of patients with schizophrenia.

Needs related to the activities of daily living are associated with the intensity of negative, disorganized and excited symptoms. Negative symptoms are also associated with socially related needs, such as handling money, relationships with other persons and lack of education. These are the type of needs that are met by day care and rehabilitation services (Saavedra et al., 2012). Van and Wiersma (2002) point out that patients with these needs benefit from rehabilitation services.

Patients' needs correlate with the current psychotic condition and severity of symptomatology rather than with the course of the disorder. This conclusion has important policy implications. In the course of any illness, services aim to help patients solve their problems (meet their needs) as soon as their psychiatric symptoms show clinical improvement or alleviation.

We found that the total number of needs correlated to patients' current level of functioning, subjective wellbeing, and psychological distress. This finding is consistent with previous prospective studies (Lasalvia et al., 2005; Slade et al., 2005) that revealed that improvement in the patients' clinical conditions and reduction in patient-rated unmet needs in the social domain predicted an increase in subjective quality of life over the follow-up period.

Summarizing, our findings suggest that the Camberwell Assessment of Need, can be useful not only for probing goals but also for appraising the quality of services and monitoring the quality of life among patients with severe mental illnesses. This is especially important in the context of current health care service reform in Israel, where the Ministry of Health is changing roles from the direct management of services to coordination, including both executive and supervision responsibilities for performance standards and the quality of care.

CONCLUSION

The frequency of needs varies substantially among need domains. There is a major gap between need for help and actual help received from services. In this chapter we described the need profile of a homogeneous group of schizophrenic patients who were hospitalized for the treatment of severe mental illness. We assessed the needs of these patients in relation to selected socio-demographic and clinical characteristics as well as to measures of their psychopathological symptoms, functioning, general wellbeing and life satisfaction. Mental health services should be provided on the basis of psychiatric patients' needs. The next chapter will familiarize the reader with psychiatric services existing in Israel in order to meet these needs.

REFERENCES

Alvarado R, Gonzalez FT, Schilling S, Alvarado F, Dominguez C, Kustner BM, Aliste F. Factors associated with unmet needs in individuals with schizophrenia in Chile. *Cad Saúde Colet* 2012, Rio de Janeiro, 20: 466-472.

American Psychiatric Association. Diagnostic and Statistical Manual of Mental Disorders, Fourth Edition: DSM-IV-TR®. *American Psychiatric Pub,* 2000, p 34.

Arikan K Uysal O. Emotional reactions to the mentally ill are positively influenced by personal acquaintance. *Isr J Psychiatry and Relat Sci* 1999;36:100-104.

Arikan K, Uysal O, Cetin G. Public awareness of the effectiveness of psychiatric treatment may reduce stigma. *Isr J Psychiatry and Relat Sci* 1999;36:95-99.

Arvidsson H. Met and unmet needs of severely mentally ill persons – the psychiatric care reform in Sweden. *Soc Psychiatry Psychiatr Epidemiol* 2003;38:373–379.

Briskman I, Bar G, Boaz M, Shargorodsky M. Impact of co-morbid mental illness on the diagnosis and management of patients hospitalized for medical conditionsin a general hospital. *Int J Psychiatry Med* 2012;43:339-348.

Bustillo J, Lauriello J, HoranW, Keith S. The psychosocial treatment of schizophrenia: an update. *Am J Psychiatry* 2001;158:163–175.

Central Bureau of Statistics.Mental Health in Israel. *Statistic Annual 2001.* Ministry of Health, Jerusalem, 2001.

Chwastiak L, Rosenheck R, Leslie D. Impact of medical comorbidity on the quality of schizophrenia pharmacotherapy in a national VA sample. *Med Care* 2006;44:55-61.

Clifford P, Charman A, Webb Y, Best S. Planning for community care.Long-stay populations of hospitals scheduled for rundown or closure. *Br J Psychiatry* 1991;158:190-196.

Davidson M. Risk of cardiovascular disease and sudden death in schizophrenia. *J Clin Psychiatry* 2002;63 Suppl 9:5-11.

Donnelly M, McGilloway S, Mays N, Perry S, Lavery C (1997) A 3- to 6-year follow-up of former long-stay psychiatric patients in Northern Ireland. *Soc Psychiatry Psychiatr Epidemiol* 32:451-458.

Druss BG, von Esenwein SA. Improving general medical care for persons with mental and addictive disorders: systematic review. *Gen Hosp Psychiatry* 2006;28:145-153.

Fakhoury WK, White I, Priebe S; PLAO Study Group. Be good to your patient: how the therapeutic relationship in the treatment of patients admitted to assertive outreach affects rehospitalization. *J Nerv Ment Dis* 2007;195:789-791.

Felker B, Yazel JJ, Short D. Mortality and medical comorbidity among psychiatric patients: a review. *Psychiatr Serv* 1996;47:1356-1363.

Foldemo A, Bogren L. Need assessment and quality of life in outpatients with schizophrenia: a 5-year follow-up study. *Scand J Caring Sci* 2002;16:393-398.

Franz M, Meyer T, Dubowy M, Hanewald B, Gallhofer B. (Accumulation of "new" long-stay patients in homes being part of psychiatric hospitals: a challenge for psychiatric care). *Psychiatr Prax* 2010;37:240-247. (in German).

Goff DC, Cather C, Evins AE, Henderson DC, Freudenreich O, Copeland PM, ierer M, Duckworth K, Sacks FM. Medical morbidity and mortality in schizophrenia: guidelines for psychiatrists. *J Clin Psychiatry* 2005;66:183-194.

Grinshpoon A, Friger M, Orev E, Shvarts S, Kaplan Z, Abramowitz MZ, Ponizovsky AM. Relative perceptions of the needs of inpatients with schizophrenia and schizoaffective disorders. *Isr J Psychiatry Relat Sci* 2008;45:201-209.

Grinshpoon A, Ponizovsky AM. The relationships between need profiles, clinical symptoms, functioning and the well-being of inpatients with severe mental disorders. *J Eval Clin Pract* 2008;14:218-225.

Grinshpoon A, Shershevsky Y, Levinson D, Ponizovsky A. Should patients with chronic psychiatric disorders remain in hospital? Results from a service inquiry. *Isr J Psychiatry Relat Sci* 2003;40:268-273.

Grinshpoon A, Zilber N, Lerner Y, Ponizovsky AM. Impact of a rehabilitation legislation on the survival in the community of long-term patients discharged from psychiatric hospitals in Israel. *Soc Psychiatry Psychiatr Epidemiol* 2006;41:87-94.

Guo X, Zhai J, Liu Z, Fang M, Wang B, Wang C, Hu B, Sun X, Lv L, Lu Z, Ma C,He X, Guo T, Xie S, Wu R, Xue Z, Chen J, Twamley EW, Jin H, Zhao J. Effect of antipsychotic medication alone vs combined with psychosocial intervention on outcomes of early-stage schizophrenia: A randomized, 1-year study. *Arch Gen Psychiatry* 2010;67:895-904.

Hamden A, Newton R, McCauley-Elsom K, Cross W. Is deinstitutionalization working in our community? *Int J Ment Health Nurs* 2011;20:274-283.

Hansson L, Bjorkman T, Svensson B. The assessment of needs in psychiatric patients.Interrater reliability of the Swedish version of the Camberwell Assessment of Needs instrument and results from a cross-sectional study. *Acta Psychiatr Scand* 1995;92:285–293.

Hansson L, Sandlund M, Bengtsson-Tops A, Bjarnason O, Karlsson H, Mackeprang T, Merinder L, Nilsson L, Sorgaard K, Vinding H, Middelboe T. The relationship of needs and quality of life in persons with schizophrenia living in the community.A Nordic multi-center study. *Nord J Psychiatry* 2003;57:5-11.

Hendrickson E.L., M.S. Schmal, and S.C. Ekleberry. *A Handbook for Mental Health and Substance Abuse Professionals.* The Haworth Press, 2004.

Holloway F. Community psychiatric care: from libertarianism to coercion.Moral panic and mental health policy in Britain. *Health Care Anal* 1996;4:35-243.

Issakidis C, Teesson M. Measurement of need for care: a trial of the Camberwell Assessment of Need and the health of the nation outcome scales. *Aust N Z J Psychiatry* 1999;33:754–759.

Landis JR, Koch GG. The measurement of observer agreement for categorical data. *Biometrics* 1977;33:159-174.

Lasalvia A, Boggian I, Bonetto C, Saggioro V, Piccione G, Zanoni C, Cristofalo D, Lamonaca D. Multiple perspectives on mental health outcome: needs for care and service satisfaction assessed by staff, patients and family members. *Soc Psychiatry Psychiatr Epidemiol* 2012;47:1035-1045.

Lasalvia A, Bonetto C, Malchiodi F, Salvi G, Parabiaghi A, Tansella M, Ruggeri M. Listening to patients' needs to improve their subjective quality of life. *Psychol Med* 2005;35:1655-1665.

Lasalvia A, RuggeriM, MazziMA, Dall'Agnola RB. The perception of needs for care in staff and patients in community-based mental health services.The South-Verona Outcome Project 3. *Acta Psychiatr Scand* 2000;102:366–375.

Leese M, Johnson S, Slade M, Parkman S, Kelly F, Phelan M, Thornicroft G. User perspective on needs and satisfaction with mental health services. PRiSM Psychosis Study 8. *Br J Psychiatry* 1998;173:409-415.

Lehman AF, Dixon L, Hoch JS, Deforge B, Kernan E, Frank R. Cost-effectiveness of assertive community treatment for homeless persons with severe mental illness. *Br J Psychiatry* 1999;174:346-352.

Lelliott P, Wing J. A national audit of new long-stay psychiatric patients. II: Impact on services. *Br J Psychiatry* 1994;165:170-178.

Leung A, Chue P. Sex differences in schizophrenia, a review of the literature. *Acta Psychiatr Scand Suppl* 2000;401:3-38.

Levinson D, Karger CJ, Haklai Z. Chronic physical conditions and use of health services among persons with mental disorders: results from the Israel National Health Survey. *Gen Hosp Psychiatry* 2008;30:226-232.

Macpherson R, Varah M, Summerfield L, Foy C, Slade M. Staff and patient assessments of need in an epidemiologically representative sample of patients with psychosis--staff and patient assessments of need. *Soc Psychiatry Psychiatr Epidemiol* 2003;38:662-667.

Majumder I, White JM, Irvine RJ.Antidepressant-like effects of ecstasy in subjects with a predisposition to depression. *Addict Behav* 2012;37:1189-1192.

Mangen S, Brewin CR. The measurement of need. In: *Social Psychiatry. Theory, Methodology and Practice* (ed. P. Bebbington). London: Transaction Publishers, 1991, pp. 162–182.

McCann E. Investigating mental health service user views regarding sexual and relationship issues. *J Psychiatr Ment Health Nurs* 2010a;17: 251-259.

McCann E. The sexual and relationship needs of people who experience psychosis: quantitative findings of a UK study. *J Psychiatr Ment Health Nurs* 2010b;17:295-303.

McCrone P, Leese M, Thornicroft G, Schene A, Knudsen HC, Vazquez-Barquero JL, Tansella M, Becker T. A comparison of needs of patients with schizophrenia in five European countries: the EPSILON Study. *Acta Psychiatr Scand* 2001;103:370-379.

Meesters PD, Comijs HC, Dröes RM, de Haan L, Smit JH, Eikelenboom P, Beekman AT, Stek ML. The care needs of elderly patients with schizophrenia spectrum disorders. *Am J Geriatr Psychiatry* 2013;21:129-137.

Merinder L-B. Patient education in schizophrenia: a review. *Acta Psychiatr Scand* 2000;102:98-106.

Middelboe T, Mackeprang T, Hansson L, Werdelin G, Karlsson H, Bjarnason O, Bengtsson-Tops A, Dybbro J, Nilsson LL, Sandlund M, Sorgaard KW. The Nordic Study on schizophrenic patients living in the community. Subjective needs and perceived help. *Eur Psychiatry* 2001;16:207-214.

Mueser KT, Deavers F, Penn DL, Cassisi J. Psychosocial Treatments for Schizophrenia. *Annu Rev Clin Psychol* 2013;9:465-497.

Nordentoft M, Øhlenschlaeger J, Thorup A, Petersen L, Jeppesen P, Bertelsen M. Deinstitutionalization revisited: a 5-year follow-up of a randomized clinical trial of hospital-based rehabilitation versus specialized assertive intervention (OPUS) versus standard treatment for patients with first-episode schizophrenia spectrum disorders. *Psychol Med* 2010;40:1619-1626.

Ochoa S, Haro JM, Usall J, Autonell J, Vicens E, Asensio F; NEDES group. Needs and its relation to symptom dimensions in a sample of outpatients with schizophrenia. *Schizophr Res* 2005;75:129-134.

Overall JE, Gorham DR (1962).The brief psychiatric rating scale. *Psychol Rep* 1962;10:799-812.

Pharoah F, Mari J, Rathbone J, Wong W. Family intervention for schizophrenia. *Cochrane Database Syst Rev* 2010;(12):CD000088.

Phelan M, Slade M, Thornicroft G et al. The Camberwell Assessment of Need (CAN): the validity and reliability of an instrument to assess the needs of the seriously mentally ill. *Br J Psychiatry* 1995;167:589–595.

Ponizovsky A, Grinshpoon A, Sasson R, Baidani-Auerbach A, Ben Eliezer D, Shershevsky Y. Knowledge and attitudes about mental disorders among principals of adult education schools. *Isr J Psychiatry and Relat Sci* 2003;40:283-289.

Rector NA, Beck AT. Cognitive therapy for schizophrenia: from conceptualization to intervention. *Can J Psychiatry* 2002;47:39-48.

Ritsner MS, Grinshpoon A. Ten-year quality of life outcomes of patients with schizophrenia and schizoaffective disorders. *Clin Schizophr Relat Psychoses* 2013;14:1-32.

Ruggeri M, Leese M, Slade M, Bonizzato P, Fontecedro L, Tansella M. Demographic, clinical, social and service variables associated with higher needs for care in community psychiatric service patients. The South Verona Outcome Project 8. *Soc Psychiatry Psychiatr Epidemiol* 2004;39:60-68.

Saavedra J, Cubero M, Crawford P. Everyday life, culture, and recovery: carer experiences in care homes for individuals with severe mental illness. *Cult Med Psychiatry* 2012;36:422-441.

Scott D, Burke K, Williams S, Happell B, Canoy D, Ronan K. Increased prevalence of chronic physical health disorders in Australians with diagnosed mental illness. *Aust N Z J Public Health* 2012;36:483-486.

Shepherd G. System failure? The problems of reductions in long-stay beds inthe UK. *Epidemiol Psichiatr Soc* 1998;7:127-134.

Slade M, Leese M, Cahill S, Thornicroft G, Kuipers E. Patient-rated mental health needs and quality of life improvement. *Br J Psychiatry* 2005;187:256-261.

Slade M, Leese M, Taylor R, Thornicroft G. The association between needs and quality of life in an epidemio epidemiologically representative sample of people with psychosis. *Acta Psychiatr Scand* 1999;100:49–57.

Slade M, Phelan M, Thornicroft G, Parkman S. The Camberwell Assessment of Need (CAN): Comparison of assessments by staff and patients of the needs of the severely mentally ill. *Soc Psychiatry Psychiatr Epidemiol* 1996;31:109–113.

Slade M, Phelan M, Thornicroft G. A comparison of needs assessed by staff and by an epidemiologically representative sample of patients with psychosis. *Psychol Med* 1998;28:543–550.

Slade M. Needs assessment. Involvement of staff and users will help to meet needs. *Br J Psychiatry* 1994;165:293–296.

Stevens A, Gabbay J. *Needs assessment, needs assessment. Health Trends* 1991;23:20-23.

Teesson M, Mitchell PB, Deady M, Memedovic S, Slade T, Baillie A. Affective and anxiety disorders and their relationship with chronic physical conditions in Australia: findings of the 2007 National Survey of Mental Health and Wellbeing. *Aust N Z J Psychiatry* 2011;45:939-946.

Thompson AH, Stuart H, Bland R, Arboleda-Flórez J, Warner R, Dickson RA. Attitudes about schizophrenia form the pilot site of the WPA worldwide campaign against the stigma of schizophrenia, *Soc Psychiatry Psychiatr Epidemiol* 2002: 37:475-482.

Thornicroft G, Gooch C, Dayson D. The TAPS project. 17: Readmission to hospital for long term psychiatric patients after discharge to the community. *BMJ* 1992;305:996-998.

Usall J, Haro JM, Ochoa S, Ma´rquez M, Araya S, and the NEDES group. Influence of gender in social outcome in schizophrenia. *Acta Psychiatr Scand* 2002;106,337–342.

Van BJ, Wiersma D. Does rehabilitation met the needs of care and improve the quality of life of patients with schizophrenia or other chronic mental disorders? *Community Ment Health J* 2002;38:61–70.

Wennstrom E, Sorbom D, Wiesel FA. Factor structure in the Camberwell Assessment of Need. *Br J Psychiatry* 2004;185:505-510.

World Health Organization. International classification of impairments, disabilities and handicaps.WHO, Geneva, 1980.

Wiersma D, Van Busschbach J. Are needs and satisfaction of care associated with quality of life? An epidemiological survey among the severely mentally ill in the Netherlands. *Eur Arch Psychiatry Clin Neurosci* 2001;251:239–246.

Wiersma D. Needs of people with severe mental illness. *Acta Psychiatr Scand* 2006;113(Suppl. 429):115–119.

Wing JK, Brewin CR, Thornicroft G. Defining mental health needs. In Thornicroft G (Ed.), Measuring mental health needs. *RCPsych Publications*, 2001, pp. 1 - 21.

Woollcott M. Access to primary care services for homeless mentally ill people. *Nurs Stand* 2008;22:40-44.

Xia J, Merinder LB, Belgamwar MR. Psychoeducation for schizophrenia. *Cochrane Database Syst Rev* 2011;(6):CD002831.

Zahid MA, Ohaeri JU. Clinical and psychosocial factors associated with needs for care: an Arab experience with a sample of treated community-dwelling persons with schizophrenia. *Soc Psychiatry Psychiatr Epidemiol* 2013;48:313-323.

Chapter 4

MENTAL HEALTH SERVICES IN ISRAEL

ABSTRACT

Effective treatment for severe mental disorders begins with the organization of services. Most mental disorders require multidisciplinary interventions including medical and psychosocial services. The delivery system of the various components impacts treatment outcome (Goldman, 1998a). It is crucial for individuals with severe mental illness to have access to mental health services, not only in order to treat symptoms but to enable participation in community life. Effective service delivery includes integrated community-based services, continuum of care by service providers, and culturally sensitive and high-quality empowering services. Service user involvement in policy and service reform, promotion of user priorities, and enabling partnerships to effect these priorities is essential for facilitating rehabilitation (Lehman and Steinwachs, 1998; Kleintjes et al., 2012). Support from the local social welfare system in the form of housing, job opportunities, welfare, and transportation is also crucial to effective service delivery (Goldman, 1998b; U.S. Department of Health and Human Services, 1999). Beginning with psychiatric hospitalization services, in this chapter we will present various mental health services available in Israel that ultimately promote integration of persons with mental illness related disabilities into the community.

PSYCHIATRIC HOSPITALIZATION

In Israel, when community based treatment does not meet the patient needs, psychiatric inpatient or day care is available in accord with the severity of the patient's illness and level of need for treatment. There are twelve psychiatric hospitals, including 8 government operated mental health centers, two mental health centers owned and operated by Clalit Health Services and two privately owned and operated psychiatric hospitals. In addition, there are nine psychiatric wards in general hospitals.

The Mental Health Treatment Act of 1955 and its 1991 amendments require that all psychiatric hospitalizations and discharges be reported to the Ministry of Health. Since the mid-1950s, the Mental Health Services at the Israel Ministry of Health has maintained a national psychiatric inpatient care database in which admissions, discharges, legal status of the admission (i.e., voluntary or compulsory, civil or criminal) and the type of hospitalization (i.e., inpatient care or day care) in all psychiatric facilities are recorded.

Demographic data are updated yearly using the National Psychiatric Case Register (NPCR). In 2011, there were 4,519 first-time admissions to inpatient or day care mental health treatment facilities in Israel. (The database does not include information about psychiatric hospitalizations outside of Israel, so a first psychiatric hospitalization in Israel does not preclude prior hospitalizations abroad.)

According to the NPCR, the rate of psychiatric hospitalizations continues to decline; 0.46 per 1000 population at the end of 2010 compared to 0.82 at the end of 2000, almost two-fold decline. The rate of first admissions at the end of 2010 was 0.59 per 1000 population that is a steady decline in first admissions since 2006. The rate of first hospitalizations at age 65 and over declined 29% since the year 2000, and continues to decline. Since the year 2000, the rate of all hospitalization among 65+ years olds has declined by 75%, in the 45-64 year old age group the rate declined by 50% and in the group age 45 or younger the rate declined by one third. During the nineties, the rate of psychiatric hospitalization was highest for 65 year olds and older, however since the year 2000 the highest rate is in the 45-64 year old age group.

In accordance with the Ministry of Health's mental health policy, the number of psychiatric hospital beds continues to be reduced. At the end of 2011 there were 3,459 beds of which 81% were in government hospitals, 10% in Clalit Health Services hospitals. About half of the beds are in active psychiatric wards and a third in chronic active departments. This compares to 5,430, in 2004, when the proportion of psychiatric beds in government-owned facilities was 68.9%.

In 2011 there were twice as many men as women aged 45-64 in psychiatric hospitals, and 2.5 as many men as women in the age range 25-44.

From age 65 and above rates of psychiatric hospitalization are comparable for men and women.

There were 1.2 million hospitalization days in 2011, about 75% in government hospitals and 8% in psychiatric departments in general hospitals. The rate of hospitalization days continues to decline: in 2011 there were 158 days per 1000 population, compared to 294 days per 1000 population in the year 2000, 407 in 1995 and 922 in 1968.

The average duration of hospital stay has declined since the 1970's. In 2010 average duration of hospitalization was 49 days compared to 47 days in 2009, 233 in the year 2000, 204 in 1995 and 189 in 1985. Duration of hospitalization is highest in private hospitals, and lowest in government and public hospitals. Especially low rates of duration of stay were recorded in psychiatric wards in general hospitals (Ministry of Health, 2012).

PSYCHIATRIC REHABILITATION

Israel's Rehabilitation in the Community of Persons with Mental Disabilities Law (RMD) was enacted in 2000 (Sefer Hakhukim, 2000). It aimed to shift the locus of treatment and care from psychiatric institutions to the community.

The RMD law stipulates that individuals are entitled to psychiatric rehabilitation services based on defined eligibility criteria and professional assessment of need. The RMD law strives to advance rehabilitation and integration into the community of persons with psychiatric disabilities by empowering them to achieve functional independence and the best possible quality of life (Rehabilitation of the Mentally Disabled in the Community Law, 2000; Shershevsky, 2006). The law entitles persons 18 years old or older, to apply for psychiatric rehabilitation services, if their mental health disability is 40% or higher on the basis of Israel National Insurance Institute criteria. Applicants who are approved by a District Rehabilitation Committee, which is composed of three mental health professionals, are eligible for services. The District Rehabilitation Committees, directed by rehabilitation coordinators, accept referrals from professional sources, make decisions about eligibility, and, with the active participation of the client, devise a personal rehabilitation program appropriate to the client's needs. The rehabilitation coordinators monitor the implementation of the individual rehabilitation plans. At present, there are nine District Rehabilitation Committees.

Implementation of this rehabilitation reform has made a substantial contribution to government efforts to shift the locus of treatment and care from psychiatric institutions to the community (Mental Health in Israel, Statistical Annuals, 2000; 2006; 2008; 2011). According to Ministry of Finance annual budget documents for the Ministry of Health, during the last ten years the proportion of funds for rehabilitation services increased from 4% to 25% of the government's total mental health budget. The decrease in rates of psychiatric hospitalization correlates with the development and implementation of psychiatric rehabilitation services in the community (Aviram et al., 2012).

In a special meeting of the social and financial cabinet, headed by Knesset Member Dr. Yuval Steinetz, approved the Mental Health Reform submitted by the Deputy Minister of Health, Knesset Member Yakov Litzman, in accord with the Treasury Department. Within the framework of the Reform, responsibility for Mental Health Services will be transferred to the various Health Funds and will be integrated in the physical health services that are under the auspices of the Health Funds. The cost of the basket of services transferred to the Health Funds is valued at over one and a half billion New Israeli Shekels (NIS), and the budget increase to expand the services is expected to amount to over 300 million NIS.

To allow the Health Funds of optimally prepare for the transfer of responsibility in the field of mental health, it was decided that funds, financed by the state will immediately begin to gradually provide mental health services to their members, until the final date of transfer which was set for July 2015 (Ministry of Health, 2013).

REHABILITATION SERVICES

The range of rehabilitation services provided includes: housing, vocational rehabilitation, supported education, peer support services, home care services, social and leisure-time activity, case management, assistance in funding dental care and the provision of information about the rehabilitation services system.

Housing services — hostels and sheltered housing—the *hostel* is for individuals who need intensive 24-hour assistance and support. There are approximately 20 residents in each hostel. The professional staff works with residents on an individual and/or group basis according to rehabilitation programs designed to promote the residents' personal, instrumental and social daily living skills in order to achieve personal autonomy.

Hostels are divided into three levels: *basic, extended-support, and comprehensive*. There is also a hostel for young adults 18-25 years old. *Basic* and *extended-support_hostels* are for residents with higher functioning levels, many of whom eventually are able to move into sheltered-housing.

Individuals with low levels of functioning but who do not require inpatient care are in *Comprehensive hostels*.

Sheltered housing is for residents who are capable of living in the community with a high degree of autonomy (usually in rented apartments), but who need regular assistance and/or support in particular aspects of daily life. The support services include regular visits, supervision and the assistance of a resident house mother/father, and the support/assistance of a mental health professional. Residents learn to manage their daily needs and achieve autonomy through the use of community institutions and resources. Residents are taught to manage money, keep house, shop, get along with neighbors and participate in leisure activities. They receive assistance in learning to improve their relationships and interactions with family and friends. Supported housing services are grouped into three levels according to the degree of residents' level of need and corresponding professional support provided.

Skills training programs prepare recovering individuals to rejoin the work force. The next stage is sheltered employment workshops where the recoveries are in a more supportive work setting, because they are not yet ready to cope with the open labor market. In the sheltered workshops they learn the vocational and social skills and behaviors that will enable them to progress into ordinary work settings. The next stage is in supported workshops which are the last stage before applying for employment in the general work force. Such employment may be designed either as a long- or short-term arrangement that will end as soon as the individual is ready for employment in the open market. The conditions of employment are guided by rehabilitation goals rather than by usual employer-employee relations. Persons undergoing rehabilitation in supported workshops receive support from rehabilitation professionals, who also maintain an ongoing relationship with the employer. Wage levels are set by agreement between the referring agency and the person undergoing rehabilitation, with the approval of the placement officer.

Peer support services are one-on-one assistance to persons recovering from mental illness, who are in the early stages of re-entry into the community. Peer companions accompany and provide support to recovering patients as they take their first steps toward integration into rehabilitation programs and other community settings.

Home care services are individual care services provided to a user in his/her home when they are in the first stage of adjustment to autonomous life in the community. The services are normally provided for 3-6 months.

Social and leisure activity services are based on the programs offered in about 60 different social clubs located throughout the country. These clubs function in the afternoon hours and provide opportunities socialization, social support and learning social skills crucial to overcoming the social isolation that individuals with mental disorders typically experience.

SERVICE ACTIVITIES

The trend toward empowering persons recovering from mental illness and facilitating integration into the community has continued to gather momentum during recent years. Considerable emphasis was placed on accelerating entry into supported housing, through the development of group-living settings designed for persons who find it difficult to live in apartments with only two or three residents. Additional occupational rehabilitation facilities were created. Social and leisure activities services were broadened through the expansion of the *Amitim* program, developed in coordination with neighborhood community centers. In the framework of this program, persons recovering from mental illness can choose between a social club for persons in a similar situation to their own, or a regular neighborhood community center, where volunteers facilitate their integration. Currently, about 615 users enjoy the services of about 25 community centers and further expansion of this program is expected. In the area of supported education services, about 500 persons recovering from mental illness attended special courses and courses leading to a high school graduation certificate (45 of the 500 attended regular community settings) and approximately 25 professionals were trained as tutors for these students. In addition, an agreement was signed between the Ministry of Health, the National Insurance Institute, the Department of Special Services and the *Re'ut* Association for a project to provide ongoing support for persons recovering from mental illness, who have been accepted by the general criteria for study in academic institutions, but who are likely to need special support and guidance during the course of their studies. Finally, it was decided to encourage the employment of persons with psychiatric disabilities by all community rehabilitation facilities, with the goal of 10% of the work force in these facilities to be persons with psychiatric disabilities.

In order to demonstrate the effectiveness of the rehabilitation programs, we conducted three studies concerning supported housing, supported education, and supported employment.

SUPPORTED HOUSING: SHOULD PATIENTS WITH CHRONIC PSYCHIATRIC DISORDERS STAY IN HOSPITAL?

Previous studies have shown that only 20-30% of persons diagnosed with schizophrenia may lead relatively normal lives, while 20-40% have persistent moderate symptoms and 40-60% significant lifelong impairments (McIntyre and Simpson, 1995; Olfson and Mechanic D, 1996). These data, coupled with a pre-reform ideology, might suggest that a substantial group of our deinstitutionalized population will be rehospitalized at some point during their community residence. The question arises as to whether or not it is justified to transfer the long-stay inpatients to community-based residences from the point of view of reducing unnecessary hospital stay and related cost-savings for the Ministry of Health. To answer this question the authors examined the reduction of inpatient days in a sample of former inpatients by calculating the proportion of subjects who were rehospitalized during their community residence and their mean hospital stay before and following placement in the hostels (Grinshpoon et al., 2003). In addition, other correlates of rehospitalization, such as gender, age, and length of hostel residence were evaluated.

The data analyzed from the NPCR that includes basic demographic and clinical information on all psychiatric hospital admissions and discharges since 1950, and an administrative database containing information on hostel residents. Fifty seven hostels participated in the study, with an average of 22 residents in each hostel. The length of follow-up period varied from 4 to 53 months.

The sample included 1,448 former long-term psychiatric inpatients that were relocated to community hostels (N=1077) or alternative community settings (N=371) between years of 1996 -1999. The cumulative length of lifetime hospitalizations of these patients ranged from 6.8 years (N=884, or 61% of the full sample) to 54.8 years (N=11, or 0.7% of the sample). A total of 797 were males and 651 were females, with a mean age of 46.9 years (range=18-65 years). The sample was divided into two groups: 1) patients that were rehospitalized during their hostel residence (hospitalized group)

(N=524), and 2) patients that did not require hospitalization (non-hospitalized group) (N=924). In the analysis (see below), we contrasted these two groups.

Of the 1448 psychiatric long-term inpatients referred to the hostels between 1996 and 1999, 524 (36.2%) were rehospitalized at some point of their hostel residence, while 924 (63.8%) were not. Overall, the rehospitalized hostel residents stayed a total of 82,718 days as inpatients. During the equivalent pre-hostel period, they stayed a total of 238,163 days. There was an average of 69 less inpatient days per patient per year that resulted in a total of 36,051 less inpatient days per year.

Was it thus justified to transfer the long stay patients to hostels? Admittedly, our inquiry was restricted to readmissions and did not examine other variables, such as changes in functioning or in quality of life, which was reported to be higher in community settings (Olfson and Mechanic, 1996; Browne et al., 1996, Heslegrave et al., 1997; Leff and Trieman 2000) than in psychiatric inpatient units (Ritsner et al., 2000). Our examination focused solely on the question whether the hostel residents required hospitalization, and if they did, how did the length of the hospital stay differ from the equivalent pre-hostel periods? Only one out of three residents was rehospitalized, and whenever hospitalization was needed, the inpatient stay was substantially shorter.

Given that the hospitalized residents tended to be an average of four years younger at first-in-life hospitalization and an average of ten years younger at the time of placement in the hostels than their non-hospitalized counterparts, one may conclude that the discharge from hospital of this group was somewhat premature. It has been reported that the earlier age of onset, the more severe the disorder is in terms of severity of psychopathology, course and outcome (Ram et al., 1992). Furthermore, young people in the early phases of a psychosis are more unstable (Gooch and Leff, 1996), and, might therefore require more frequent or prolonged hospitalizations than older people. This does not imply, however, that they should remain inpatients. Indeed, our findings show that even for these individuals with more severe illness, there was a meaningful reduction in inpatient days after placement in the hostels compared to their equivalent pre-hostel period.

We found that rehospitalized patients who entered the hostels 13-24 months prior to the follow-up had significantly shorter duration of hospitalizations than those with longer or shorter residences in the hostels. The effects of gender, age, and time spent in hostel on length of rehospitalizations warrant further investigation.

Limitations of this study Include selection bias which is a common limitation of retrospective database studies. The use of utilization-based measures such as readmission rates and length of inpatient stay should be approached with caution because these single-outcome measures do not reflect other important aspects of community-based residence of former long-stay inpatients.

At the time the study was performed, readmission to a psychiatric hospital was the only available option to provide the care needed for the hostel residents during an emergency. This study did show, however, that the vast majority of former psychiatric inpatients transferred to community-based settings could function without hospitalization.

SUPPORTED EDUCATION

Education is an essential stepping stone to employment in western society. Supported education programs help people with mental illness to obtain the basic academic skills necessary to pursue post high school education and employment (Gutman et al., 2007). Because the onset of mental illness is generally in late adolescence and early adulthood, many people with psychiatric disabilities have failed to obtain college or other post high school degrees that lead to employment (Mowbray et al., 2005). Consequently, individuals with mental illness frequently have gaps in their basic education and they often lack the interpersonal skills necessary to succeed in the student or worker role (Gutman et al., 2009). For those with the onset of mental illness later in adult life, re-training may be necessary to prepare them for alternate career directions (Stoneman and Lysagh, 2010).

Supported education is the service provided to help individuals with mental disorders gain access to and succeed in a post high school educational programs such as college or technical school. Recovery-oriented programs aim to empower individuals to live independently in the community and overcome the stigma of being perceived as mental patients. Supported education can thus be considered one of the most important tools for recovery as it offers individuals with psychiatric disabilities the opportunity return to educational institutions as students to prepare themselves for the professional world of job and career advancement.

To promote recovery and facilitate the successful relocation of individuals with psychiatric disabilities to the community, The Mental Health Services at Israel's Ministry of Health, now focusses on the potential of supported education. Studies across the globe have shown that supported education for this target group not only provides useful schooling but contributes significantly to general rehabilitation goals by opening a new avenue for the rehabilitation of persons with mental-illness-related disability (Unger, 2010; Mowbray et al., 2005; Gutman et al., 2009). It gives those who enroll something to aim for, sets realistic objectives and helps repair a damaged self-image. Supported education also helps counteract the public stigma suffered by the mentally disabled and their own pessimism about their ability to integrate into community services.

SUPPORTED EDUCATION AS A COMPONENT OF REHABILITATION

Anthony and Liberman (1986) define rehabilitation as a process teaching the emotional, instrumental and intellectual skills needed for living, learning and working in the community. Education and training are perceived as important and necessary sources of the sense of being in charge of one's own life: they open up the possibility of using knowledge-dependent tools, provide a sense of ability and progress, and are important factors in the respect people get from others and give themselves. Learning is the key to the ability to define new goals, behaviors and life content for oneself.

Frankie et al (1996) noted the reasons that impede individuals with mental disabilities from attaining higher education, with emphasis on the obstacles within the educational settings themselves, where the mentally disabled are exposed to stigma and discrimination. However researchers have found that mental disability in itself is not the reason for lack of participation in normative educational settings and meeting the required goals and achievement level, as long as specially designed syllabuses are made available and include both an appropriate academic program and supportive administrative services. Individuals with mental disability, who become involved in planning and implementing courses of study, also benefit from increased self-esteem and encouragement to join such programs in the future.

In an overview of supported education, Soydan (2004) declared that the essence of supported education is the process of psychiatric rehabilitation, with its unique client-centered focus of individualized goal setting and readiness, skill, and support assessments; and personalized skill and resource development. In addition, he suggested that supported education might go beyond rehabilitation to assist in the process of recovery and play a key role in providing new and powerful opportunities for people who are in the process of adjusting to psychiatric disability and trying to move beyond its pervasive impact.

Various unique supported education programs have been established in different countries. Stoneman and Lysaght (2010) described a specialized retail sales training program targeting the needs of individuals with mental health concerns. An existing retail workforce curriculum served as the basis for the program, and was adapted to meet the needs of students with mental disabilities. The curriculum was also modified to comply with the standards set by the College Academic and Career Entrance Certificate (ACE) Self-Management/Self Direction course, such that this certification could be awarded to successful trainees. An instructor with 20 years' retail experience who had previously provided vocational skills training to clients was hired as the primary course instructor. There were 12 weeks of daily classroom instruction, and a 3 week community work placement. Skills for Retail have since been offered three times and 20 out of 29 participants who completed the program are still employed (length of employment ranging from 6 to 24 months). Considering the significant barriers to employment encountered people with psychiatric disabilities these results are encouraging for people who are struggling with mental illness (Stoneman and Lysaght, 2010).

McDiarmid et al (2005) described e Consumer as Provider (CAP) Training program at the University of Kansas - School of Social Welfare, which creates opportunities for individuals with severe psychiatric disabilities to develop knowledge and skills to be effective as human service providers. CAP fosters a partnership between colleges and community mental health centers where students experience classroom and internship activities. Outcome from a 2-year longitudinal study on CAP graduates indicates increased employability, especially in social services field, and higher post-secondary educational involvement.

Shor and Avihod (2011) described an innovative culturally-oriented supported-education program that was established in Israel to address the needs of religious Jewish persons with severe mental illness. This program utilized a highly respected institution in the Orthodox communities, a Beit Midrash, a study hall for religious studies, as a context for rehabilitation. Common principles of psychiatric rehabilitation were adapted and incorporated into this novel context for psychiatric rehabilitation. Innovative supported-education methods that are compatible with the cultural context of Orthodox Jewish persons were implemented, including opportunities to reconstruct their views of their daily struggles and enhance their sense of spirituality via the discussion of socially-oriented religious texts. The culturally-oriented context of the Beit Midrash promoted outreach to the Orthodox Jewish population which might otherwise not receive adequate services. This is a promising supported education model for addressing the unique needs of religious people with severe mental illness and for filling a gap in the resources available for the rehabilitation of this population in the community.

Rehabilitation Programs

Following a three stage process of (defining policy, defining the target population and its needs, and design and implementation of the intervention program), supported education is now included in the basket of services offered to the mentally disabled in Israel. By law, mentally disabled individuals can receive financial support to complete their education including Hebrew language classes (for recent immigrants), elementary and high school education, and computer skills training (Sasson et al., 2005).

Defining Policy

Policy includes identification of the target population's special education needs; assessment of the potential of available educational settings to contribute to the supported education service; integration of the contributions of the health, education and immigrant absorption systems; identification and training suitable teachers and establishment of performance standards and guidelines, determination of evaluation indicators; de- and implementation of quality assurance mechanisms and an ongoing report system to the Ministry of Health's Information and Evaluation Center.

Defining the Target Population and its Needs

The Ministry of Health's Information and Evaluation Center provided the data regarding the level of education of inpatients for the given year. For 6,016 out of the 12,224 persons aged 21-55 who had been mental inpatients at least one day in 1998 the Center was able to furnish their total number of years of schooling. No schooling data was available for the other half of the population:

The data showed that over half the population had more than twelve years of schooling, thus the intervention was expected to provide a high level of diverse services to a high level to meet the needs of groups with various levels of education. The ability of each candidate to study and learn, as reported by their personal carer also needed to be considered.

Within the 6,016 mentally disabled persons listed above, approximately 4,500 (75%) were new immigrants, of whom 15% arrived after 1994 and needed Hebrew language classes.

The Program Designed and Implemented, 1998-2000

In order to design programs appropriate for the potential participants, questionnaires were sent to the professional carers in community clinics, employment centers and social clubs for the mentally ill in which they were requested to as their clients what gaps in their education they wished to fill. 440 questionnaires were returned, and 180 of the respondents had adequate schooling to be considered suitable candidates for intervention. These potential participants were allocated by area of residence, years of schooling and level of need to 10 adult education colleges around the country, where their classroom work was intensively supported by professional carers from outside the college. Evaluation questionnaires were filled out by all students at the beginning of the intervention to provide baseline data on self-esteem, mental problems, coping with pressure, and the need for social support. There were three months of classes (72 hours) in subjects from computer familiarization through reading comprehension, citizenship and Bible studies. At the end of the three months, college deans and teachers, outside carers, representatives of the Mental Health Services, and a representative of the Israeli National Insurance Institution (where the INII had helped fund tuition fees) met to assess the educational and rehabilitation achievements of each student and to draw conclusions regarding continuation of the intervention.

Rehabilitees who completed their Introduction to Computing course are now are now employed by Enosh (the Israeli advocacy association for the mentally disabled) in secretarial positions, and others found employment typing dissertation and seminar papers for students in Rishon Lezion. In addition to their educational achievements, carers reported a marked improvement in self-esteem and self-confidence of the participants, and family members reported a better family atmosphere because the students had were interested in their studies and occupations, were satisfied, happier, and were less afflicted by anxiety and hallucinations. Teachers reported that the stigma that they had previously associated with persons with psychiatric disabilities had been dispelled and that they had built positive relationships with their students. One college principal was so impressed by the students' achievements and perseverance that she decided to enroll them in regular classes the following year.

Rehabilitees who had not completed matriculation exams and who were able to join regular classes were enrolled in standard preparatory programs for matriculation examinations. These students received additional support and assistance from mental health professionals. Before classes began, we had met with the college principals and teaching supervisors to answer questions regarding the unique new student population in an attempt to dispel fear and stigma and ultimately these programs generated positive responses from both students and carers.

In the 1999/2000 school year, for new immigrants who had been in the country less than five years, we opened 30 standard Hebrew-language classes in mental health centers, hostels, and clinics, as well as in public community centers. The program was jointly organized and run by the Ministry of Education's Department of Adult Education and the Jewish Agency's Department of Immigrant Absorption, and there were 6-15 students per class. Learning Hebrew was an important step to the participants' rehabilitation.

Future Plans

- To give more persons with mental illness-related disability the opportunity to enroll in regular adult education college classes.
- With the cooperation of universities and colleges and with funding from the Israel National Insurance Institute's Special Needs Department and governmental rehabilitation services, to support the mentally disabled interested in obtaining a formal qualification and/or completing their academic education.
- To evaluate the effect of supported education on self-esteem, mental problems, coping with stress situations and the need for social support based on the information gleaned from the initial evaluation questionnaires, filled out by participants in the first intervention.

Rudnick and Gover (2009) reported on a successful project of supported education in Ra'anana, Israel. They noted that although supported employment has often had remarkable success in arranging gainful employment for individuals with serious mental illness such as schizophrenia, the success was generally in unskilled vocational occupations. They performed a pilot project that combined supported employment and supported education conducted at the vocational rehabilitation and training center in Ra'anana, Israel. The center provides certified courses in skilled occupations for individuals with various disabilities. Applicants were referred to an intake meeting conducted by the project's social worker and were then selected by a multidisciplinary staff at the center. The participants continued to receive mental health care, as needed, by their pre-project mental health care services.

Of the 53 participants who completed the first stage of training, 15 completed their course, 31 were still studying, four dropped out (one was already in supported employment), and three took a break. Of the 15 who completed their course, six were competitively employed in their vocation of choice, five were in individual training for gainful employment, two were searching for work, and two were working in sheltered (industrial) employment as a planned transition to supported employment.

Many individuals with mental illness related disabilities are capable of performing in educational settings and reaching a reasonable level of achievement as long as they have an appropriate support system. From the responses of rehabilitees, carers and family members it is clear that the supported education improves self-confidence, general functioning and the ability to cope with stress. It has been shown that the overall anxiety level drops and students feel a considerable degree of satisfaction

SUPPORTED EDUCATION PROGRAMS –
AND ASSOCIATED STRESS

The successful integration of the former psychiatric inpatients into the community requires innovative programs of psychosocial rehabilitation, including supported education. Ponizovsky et al (2004) examined psychological distress as an outcome variable, and social support and coping strategies as mediating variables among 70 service user students (SUS) with severe mental illness and 55 adult students (AS) with no psychiatric diagnosis as a comparison group that attended a supported education program. The study parameters were assessed using standardized research instruments. Univariate and multivariate analyses were used to examine the obtained data. Compared with the AS group, the SUS reported, higher emotional distress, the utilization of emotion- and avoidance-oriented coping strategies, and less friend support. In this group, the factors that were significantly associated with experiencing emotional distress were the use of emotional-oriented coping, and lack of perceived social support from friends and family. The findings provide the basis for interventions geared to reduce distress and, as a result, to enable the students with severe mental illness to fully utilize the supported education program.

Published reports of supported education evaluations show that nearly one third of mentally ill consumers' drops out of the program due to increased stress and symptomatology (Lieberman et al., 1993). Our findings suggest the need for specific interventions to help these students to prevent distress and to be sufficiently stable to fully utilize a supported education program. The focus of the interventions should be to recognize the availability of social support from family and friends, and utilization of more adaptive coping resources, such as task- and avoidance- (social distraction) oriented coping devises. Interpersonal interventions combining elements of communication training, problem solving, along with social skills training should be implemented prior to enrollment into supported education programs to prevent emotional distress and, thus, to enhance scholastic achievement and social rehabilitation in general.

SUPPORTED EMPLOYMENT

In the Supported Education Program developed in Israel (Sasson et al., 2005), a mental health team of specially trained social workers, occupational therapists, and teaching staff provides academic and emotional support to rehabilitees during their studies. They also support participants in coping with the educational environment, such as troubleshooting stress situations and introducing them to support networks; and encouraging peer support from their peers in supported education or other psychosocial rehabilitation programs (Moxley et al., 1993). Throughout the program, an educational team monitors student attendance, relationships formed at the school with peers, teacher-student communications, academic achievement, the relationship formed with professional support staff, as well as the team's response to cognitive difficulties.

Though the benefits of helping former inpatients to complete a relatively advanced study program are obvious the stumbling blocks towards that goal have not been sufficiently examined (Ponizovsky et al., 2004). Among others, social support has been recognized as a key factor in achieving educational and vocational goals (Collins et al., 2000; Ponizovsky et al., 2003).

A major obstacle to the success of a SEP is negative stigmatizing attitudes with respect to psychiatric disorders and the persons affected by them among the professionals responsible for the daily running of the programs (Corrigan et al., 2004).

Further acquaintance with SEPs has convinced us that the knowledge of and attitudes to psychiatric disorders of the mental health professionals immediately involved in the program may play an important role in the program's success. The next step, therefore, was to examine these issues among social workers employed in SEP in order to lend social and emotional support and help to the students with psychiatric disabilities.

The results suggest that the participation in the SEP can potentially foster more positive attitudes among social workers involved. This in turn would enable better integration of persons with psychiatric disabilities into the adult education system. Special psychoeducation programs designed to increase mental health knowledge and promote favorable attitudes among social workers (and probably teachers and fellow students) would benefit the rehabilitation process.

CONCLUSION

In this chapter we considered the current psychiatric services in Israel as well as research findings on supported education and employment among severe mentally ill people in the rehabilitation framework. As noted earlier in this chapter, Israel underwent the Reform of psychiatric hospitalization services, therefore in the next chapter some consequences of this changes, such as surviving patients with SMI in the community and new institutionalization will be addressed.

REFERENCES

Anthony WA, Liberman RP. The practice of psychiatric rehabilitation: historical, conceptual, and research base. *Schizophr Bull* 1986;12:542-559.

Aviram U, Ginath Y, Roe D. Mental health reforms in Europe: Israel's rehabilitation in the community of persons with mental disabilities law: challenges and opportunities. *Psychiatr Serv* 2012;63:110-112.

Browne S, Roe M, Lane A, Gervin M, Morris M, Kinsella M, Larkin A, Callaghan EO. Quality of life in schizophrenia: Relationship to sociodemographic factors, symptomatology and tardive dyskinesia. *Acta Psychiatr Scand* 1996; 94:118-124.

Collins ME, Mowbray CT, Bybee D. Characteristics predicting successful outcomes of participants with severe mental illness in supported education. *Psychiatr Serv* 2000;51:774–780.

Cook JA, Solomon ML. The community scholar program: An outcome study of supported education for students with severe mental illness. *Psychosoc Rehabil J* 1993;17: 83-97.

Frankie PA, Levine P, Mowbray CT, Shriner W, Conklin C, Thomas ER. Supported education for persons with psychiatric disabilities: Implementation in an urban setting. *J Behav Health Serv Res* 1996;23:406-417.

Goldman HH. *Organizing mental health services: An evidence-based approach.* Stockholm: Swedish Council on Technology Assessment in Health Care, 1998a.

Goldman HH. Deinstitutionalization and community care: Social welfare policy as mental health policy. *Harv Rev Psychiatry* 1998b;6:219–222.

Gooch C, Leff J. Factors affecting the success of community placement: The TAPS Project 26. *Psychol Med* 1996; 26:511-520.

Grinshpoon A, Shershevsky Y, Levinson D, Ponizovsky A. Should patients with chronic psychiatric disorders remain in hospital? Results from a service inquiry. *Isr J Psychiatry Relat Sci* 2003;40:268-273.

Gutman SA, Schindler VP, Klien K, Lisak JM, Durham D. The effectiveness of supported education program for adults with psychiatric disabilities: The bridge program. *Occup Ther Ment Health* 2007;23:23-38.

Gutman SA, Kerner R, Zombek I, Dulek J, Ramsey CA. Supported education for adults with psychiatric disabilities: effectiveness of an occupational therapy program. *Am J Occup Ther* 2009;63:245-254.

Heslegrave RJ, Awad AG, Voruganti LN. The influence of neurocognitive deficits and symptoms on the quality of life in schizophrenia. *J Psychiatry Neurosci* 1997; 22:235-243.

Kleintjes S, Lund C, Swartz L. South African mental health care service user views on priorities for supporting recovery: implications for policy and service development. *Disabil Rehabil* 2012;34:2272-2280.

Leff J, Trieman N. Long stay patients discharged from psychiatric hospitals. *Br J Psychiatry* 2000;176:217-223.

Lehman AF, Steinwachs DM. Patterns of usual care for schizophrenia: Initial results from the Schizophrenia Patient Outcomes Research Team (PORT) Client Survey. *Schizophr Bull* 1998;24:11–20.

Lieberman HJ, Goldberg FR, Jed J. Helping seriously mentally ill patients to become students. *Psychosoc Rehabil J* 1993;17:99-107.

McDiarmid D, Rapp C, Ratzlaff S. Design and initial results from a supported education initiative: the Kansas Consumer as Provider program. *Psychiatr Rehabil J* 2005;29:3-9.

McIntyre CM, Simpson GM. Schizophrenia disorders. In: Rakel RE, editor. *Conn's current therapy*. St. Louis, MO: W.B. Saunders, 1995.

Mental Health in Israel, Statistical Annuals, 2006 Jerusalem, Ministry of Health, Mental Health Services, Department of Information and Evaluation, 2006.

Mental Health in Israel, Statistical Annuals, 2008, Jerusalem, Ministry of Health, Mental Health Services, Department of Information and Evaluation, 2009.

Ministry of Health. http://www.health.gov.il/NewsAndEvents/SpokemanMessages/Pages/01052012_2.aspx

Ministry of Health, Department of Information Services. Inpatient facilities and day care hospitalization units in 2010. Ministry of Health, Jerusalem, 2011.

Mowbray CT, Collins ME, Bellamy CD, Megivern, DA., Bybee D, Szilvagyi, S. Supported education for adults with psychiatric disabilities: An innovation for social work and psychosocial rehabilitation practice. *Soc Work* 2005;50:7–20.

Mowbray CT, Collins M, Bybee, D. Supported education for individuals with psychiatric disabilities: Long-term outcomes from an experimental study. *Soc Work Res* 1999; 23:89-100.

Mowbray CT, Collins ME. The effectiveness of supported education: Current research findings. In C. T. Mowbray, K. S. Brown, K. F. Norman & A. S. Soydan (Eds.), *Supported education and psychiatric rehabilitation*. Linthicum, MD: International Association of Psychosocial Rehabilitation Services, 2002.

Moxley, D P, Mowbray CT, Brown K S. Supported education.In R. Flexer & P. Solomon (Eds.), *Psychiatric rehabilitation in practice*. New York: Butterworth, 1993, pp. 137–152.

Olfson M, Mechanic D. Mental disorders in public, private, non-profit, and proprietary general hospitals. *Am J Psychiatry* 1996; 153:1613-1619.

Ponizovsky A, Grinshpoon A, Sasson R, Baidani-Auerbach A, Ben Eliezer D, Shershevsky Y. Knowledge and attitudes about mental disorders among principals of adult education schools. *Isr J Psychiatry Relat Sci* 2003;40:283-289.

Ponizovsky A, Grinshpoon A, Sasson R, Levav I. Stress in adult students with schizophrenia in a supported education program. *Compreh Psychiatry* 2004;45:401-407.

Ponizovsky A, Shvarts S, Sasson R, Grinshpoon A. Mental health knowledge and attitudes among social workers employed in a supported education program for adult students with schizophrenia. *Am J Psychiatr Rehabil* 2008;11:279-294.

Ponizovsky A, Grinshpoon A, Sasson R, Levav I. Stress in adult students with schizophrenia in a supported education program. *Compr Psychiatry* 2004;45:401–407.

Ram R, Bromet EJ, Eaton WW, Pato C, Schwartz JE. The natural course of schizophrenia: A review of first-admission studies. *Schizophr Bull* 1992;18:185-207.

Ratzlaff S, McDiarmid D, Marty D, Rapp C. The Kansas Consumer as Provider program: measuring the effects of a supported education initiative. *Psychiatr Rehabil J* 2006;29:174-182.

Rehabilitation of the Mentally Disabled in the Community Law, 2000 Jerusalem, Ministry of Justice, 2000. Available at www.old.health.gov.il/Download/pages/lawENG040409_2.pdf

Ritsner M, Modai, I, Endicott, J, Rivkin O, Nechamkin Y, Barak P, Goldin V. Ponizovsky A. Differences in quality of life domains, psychopathaological and psychosocial factors in psychiatric patients. *J Clin Psychiatry* 2000;61:880-889.

Rudnick A, Gover M. Combining supported education with supported employment. *Psychiatr Serv* 2009;60:1690-1690.

Sasson R, Grinshpoon A, Lachman M, Ponizovsky A. A program of supported education for adult Israeli students with schizophrenia. *Psychiatr Rehabil J* 2005;29:139–141.

Sefer Hakhukim, 2000 (Book of Laws-2000), No. 1746, July 21, 2000, p. 231. (HH 2000 No. 2782, p. 222.) Entered into force six months after publication.

Shershevsky Y. Rehabilitation package of services for mentally disabled persons in the community; in Mental Health Services in Israel: Trends and Issues (in Hebrew) Edited by Aviram U; Ginath Y Tel Aviv, Cherikover, 2006.

Shor R, Avihod G. The conceptual model and guiding principles of a supported-education program for Orthodox Jewish persons with severe mental illness. *Community Ment Health J* 2011;47:568-572.

Soydan AS. Supported education: A portrait of a psychiatric rehabilitation intervention. *Am J Psychiatr Rehabil* 2004;7:227-248.

Statistical Abstract for Israel, 2000. No 51. Jerusalem, Central Bureau of Statistics, 2000.

Statistical Abstract for Israel, 2010. No 61. Jerusalem, Central Bureau of Statistics, 2010.

Stoneman J, Lysaght R. Supported education: A means for enhancing employability for adults with mental illness.Work: *J Prevent Assess Rehabil* 2010;36:257–259.

U.S. Department of Health and Human Services. Mental Health: A Report of the Surgeon General—Executive Summary. Rockville, MD: U.S. Department of Health and Human Services, Substance Abuse and Mental Health Services Administration, Center for Mental Health Services, National Institutes of Health, National Institute of Mental Health, 1999.

Unger, K, Pfaltzgraf, B, Nikkel R. A supported education program in a state psychiatric hospital. *Psychiatr Serv* 2010;61:632-632.

Chapter 5

COMMUNITY-BASED
REHABILITATION NEEDS

ABSTRACT

Deinstitutionalization is an unprecedented process of transition from care in traditional psychiatric hospitals to care in community-based facilities. The ideology behind deinstitutionalization is that "long-stay" institutionalized patients could be discharged if adequate community facilities are available, thus leading to a steep decline in the need for inpatient beds (Holloway, 1996; Clifford et al., 1991; Lelliott and Wing 1994; Vázquez-Bourgon et al., 2012). However, in many countries the dramatic reduction in the number of psychiatric beds preceded the adequate development of facilities in the community. As a result, many former psychiatric inpatients found themselves in the community, homeless and socially deprived (Scott, 1993; Forchuk et al., 2007; Hamden et al., 2011) and "new long stay" patients accumulated in psychiatric hospitals, with multiple recurrent hospitalizations (Wing, 1971; Thornicroft et al., 1992; Machado et al., 2012) and an increase in involuntary confinement (Bauer et al., 2007). To compensate for the lack of inpatient facilities new forms of institutionalization have emerged in community settings, such as supported housing with varying levels of supervision. In this chapter we will discuss the effects of the reduction of the number of psychiatric hospital beds, and how the transfer of individuals with severe mental illness promoted integration into the community or the emergence of new forms of community based institutionalization.

In Israel, the mental health reform was implemented later than in many European countries. Although the process of deinstitutionalization began in the early 80's, the Rehabilitation Law, which provides a basket of rehabilitation services for mentally disabled patients, was not implemented until 2000. Taking advantage of the negative experiences from other countries, Israel attempted to build an adequate supportive mental health infrastructure in the community prior to the massive reduction of the number of inpatient beds (from 1.17 per 1000 population in 1996 to 0.44 in 2012 – Central Bureau of Statistics).

In parallel with the reduction of psychiatric beds, the number of hostels and sheltered homes has rapidly increased: in 1996 there were 17 hostels and 1050 people in supported housing settings in the country, and in 2011 there were 110 hostels with 5,300 people in supported housing (data from the National Psychiatric Hospitalization Registry in Israel).

Before the law was implemented, only 4,600 persons participated in any rehabilitation program. After implementation of the law the number increased, reaching 16,493 in 2011. This is consistent with the fact that the annual number of hospitalized psychiatric patients increased only from 13,000 to 14,000, although the number of people with mental disabilities eligible for rehabilitation services increased from 44,000 to 59,000 between 2001 and 2007 (Hornik et al., 2012).

IMPACT OF THE ISRAELI REHABILITATION LAW ON THE OUTCOME OF DISCHARGED PATIENTS

Grinshpoon et al (2006) examined the impact of community care following the implementation of the Rehabilitation Law 2000 on the outcome of discharge of psychiatric patients from long-term hospitalization. They compared the outcomes of long-stay psychiatric inpatients discharged from a psychiatric hospital that was closed in 1997 prior to the implementation of the Rehabilitation Law to the outcomes of long-stay psychiatric inpatients discharged from a hospital that was closed in 2000, after the implementation of the law.

This was the first study that compared the outcomes of unselected cohorts of patients discharged from two long-stay psychiatric hospitals in Israel. The authors performed a naturalistic investigation to examine how the Law affected discharge to the community, continuity of residential care, readmission to psychiatric hospitals and mortality. Analyses were performed after controlling for demographic and clinical characteristics of the cohorts.

Data were extracted from the National registry of Psychiatric Hospitalizations, the general validity of which has previously been demonstrated (Lichtenberg et al., 1999; Weiser et al., 2005).

The authors found that after the implementation of the Rehabilitation Law of 2000, following the closure of psychiatric hospitals, patients were more likely to be discharged directly into the community. Readmission rates also tended to be lower for those patients who were discharged into the community after enactment of the law both for those who were discharged directly to the community and for those who were first transferred to another hospital and then to the community.

Interestingly, the Rehabilitation Law did not have a significant effect on patients' mortality after the initial discharge. Study results indicated that the Rehabilitation Law 2000 has a clear beneficial effect on the opportunities of long-stay psychiatric patients to resettle in the community, without increasing risk of death. In addition, duration of re-hospitalization was found to be affected more by hospital policy than by changes in outpatient services.

The results are consistent with findings from the TAPS project studies, that showed a generally beneficial outcome for the majority of long-stay patients discharged from two psychiatric hospitals in London, England, followed over one year (Leff et al., 1996) and five years (Leff and Trieman, 2000). They also support findings of studies of long-stay patients resettled in the community after closure of psychiatric hospitals in the USA (Rothbard et al., 1999; Desai and Rosenheck, 2003) and in Italy (Barbato et al., 2004). Findings of the above studies show that ongoing efforts to reduce inpatient hospital beds have not resulted in increased mortality rates or clinical deterioration, and that community based residence and care can improve social behavior and enhance the quality of life of former psychiatric inpatients.

Seventy percent of the residents in supported housing have a diagnosis of schizophrenia (Grinshpoon et al., 2003). Despite the benefits of community treatment, following implementation of the Law the need for acute beds for chronic patients remains.

Our data indicate that a substantial proportion of patients in community settings require transient readmissions to hospital, which creates a steady demand for acute beds. Although this proportion has significantly decreased following implementation of the Rehabilitation Law, recurrent and sporadic readmissions are inevitable for high-risk patients with schizophrenia and other chronic illnesses, regardless of their living conditions. The mean cumulative duration of hospitalization was 26.38 days per patient per year (from discharge until death or end of their follow-up period). Thus, the number of beds needed for 100 such patients on a given day is 26.38x100/365=7.23. Thus, in order to meet this demand, about 7 beds per day are required for every 100 long-stay patients discharged to the community and this should be taken into account in planning psychiatric services (Grinshpoon et al., 2006).

NEW INSTITUTIONALIZATION AS A REBOUND PHENOMENON?

Despite differences in the specific objectives and variations in the time frames of the implementation of mental health reforms in Europe, almost all countries underwent major mental health reforms that aimed at moving mental health care from psychiatric hospitals to services in the community. Community based settings that offer various levels of treatment and supervision have proliferated to serve the population of former psychiatric inpatients. New forms of institutionalized mental health care have increased significantly in European countries since 1990 (Priebe et al., 2008; Fakhoury and Priebe, 2007). In particular, there has been a substantial increase of forensic beds and placements in residential care and supported housing. Prison populations have also been rising, though changes in involuntary hospital admissions have been inconsistent and the number of psychiatric hospital beds has declined (Abramowitz et al., 2008).

'Re-institutionalization' and "transinstitutionalization" are terms that have been used to describe the increase of new d forms of institutionalized mental health care that have emerged. This may suggest a type of rebound phenomenon following the significant deinstitutionalization in the last century which might have gone too far (Abramowitz et al., 2008).

Although the increase of forensic beds and placements in residential care and supported housing initiated a debate on whether current directions of mental health policy are on the right track, the reasons for the emergence of new venues of institutionalized mental health care remain unclear. Can this tendency can be explained as an outgrowth of the shared history of most Western European countries (i.e., the establishment of large asylums in the 19th century and the subsequent wide reaching deinstitutionalization in the second half of the 20th century) or are the current trends independent of the history of mass deinstitutionalization? Abramowitz et al (2008) analyzed changes in health care provision in Israel and compared them with data reported for countries in Western Europe from 1991/2 - 2002/3 (Priebe et al., 2005).

During the decade evaluated, the number of psychiatric hospital beds in Israel was reduced by 42%, and the number of places in supported housing in the community tripled. Although the number of psychiatric beds in prisons did not change, the number of patients treated in both prison psychiatric outpatient and hospital facilities rose by 61% and 17%, respectively. Similar trends were observed in all countries compared.

A 125% increase in the number of involuntary psychiatric hospitalizations in Israel was similar to the trends reported in England, the Netherlands and Germany, but not in Spain, Italy, and Sweden, where a decline in involuntary admissions was observed during the same period.

The reduction in the number of psychiatric hospital beds might account for delay in treatment that can lead to a further deterioration of mental disorders leading to emergency situations that often ultimately require involuntary hospitalizations that perhaps could have been avoided by timely voluntary admission. Involuntary commitments increased most in countries where the number of hospital beds was rapidly reduced, such as in England (Wall et al., 1999) and Israel (Bauer et al., 2007).

Table 1. Number of forensic beds, involuntary hospital admissions, places in residential care or supported housing, psychiatric hospital beds, and prison population in mental health care in Israel and 6 Western European Nations in 1991/2 and 2002/3. Values are numbers per 100,000 population, unless stated otherwise (data of European Nations extracted from Priebe et al., 2005)

Service provision	Israel	England	Germany	Italy	Netherlands	Spain	Sweden
Forensic beds	Beds(Patients)[1]						
1990	0.98(0.47)(1991)	1.3(1991)	4.6	2.0	4.7(1991)	1.2(1992)	9.8(1993)
2002	0.98(0.55)	1.8[3](2001)	7.8	2.2(2002)	11.54	1.5	143(2001)
Change(%)	- +17	+38	+70	+10	+143	+25	+46
Involuntary admissions							
1992	50.4	40.5(1991)	114.4	20.51	16.4	33.8	39.0
2001	70/7	50.3	190.5	18.14[4]	19.1[5](1999)	31.8[6]	32.4[7]
Change(%)	+40.3	+24	+67	-12	-36	-6	-17
Places in supported housing							
1996	18.2	15.9(1997)	8.9(1990)	8.8(1992)	24.8(1992)	5.1(1994)	76.0(1997)
2003	74.0	22.3(2002)	17.9(1996)	31.6[4](2000)	43.8(2001)	12.7[6]	33.1(2002)
Change(%)	+307	+40	+101	+259	+77	+149	+15
Psychiatric hospital beds							
1990	140.5(1991)	131.8	141.7	4.5(1992)	159.2	59.5(1991)	168.6
2002	114.5(2003)	62.8(2001)	128(2000)	5.3[4](2000)	135.5(2001)	43.0(1999)	58.3(2001)
Change(%)	-18.5	-52	-10	+18	-15	-28	-65
Prison population (Outpatient care)[2] Total population							
1992	0.99	90	71	81	49	90	63
2002	1.59(2003)	141(2003)	98(2003)	100	100	136(2003)	73
Change(%)	+61	+57	+38	+23	+104	+51	+16

[1] Number of psychiatric patients in forensic wards. [2] Imprisoned psychiatric patients. [3] Data refer to restricted patients admitted to all (high security and other) hospitals. [4] Data for Emilia-Romagna, a region in northern Italy with a population of 4 million. [5] Data for Drenthe, a rural area with 450,000 inhabitants. [6] Data for Andalucia, the second largest region in Spain, with a population of 7 million. [7] Discharges from treatment under the Compulsory Care Act during a six month period.

Reprinted from Abramowitz M, Grinshpoon A, Priebe S, Ponizovsky AM. New institutionalization as a rebound phenomenon? The case of Israel. *Isr J Psychiatry Relat Sci*.2008;45:272-277 (with permission).

Though increased involuntary commitment increased in England, the Netherlands, and Germany, it did not increase in Spain, Italy, and Sweden. This might result from different perspectives on medico-legal issues in different countries, such as the recommended psychiatric risk-management of the marginally dangerous patient not in an institutionalized setting. Finally, the possibility of comorbidity with psychoactive substance abuse and mental illness may cause an increase in involuntary admissions in some countries and a reduction in others.

In Israel, mental health reform with initiatives to establish services in the community came relatively late, legislation was passed in 2000 (Grinshpoon et al., 2006).

The disproportionate increase in supported housing in Israel within one decade might reflect the search for alternative solutions to hospitalization, transfer of responsibility for difficult patients to the social welfare services. The comparison among the various countries revealed that those countries with a relatively high baseline figure in 1990 for supported housing, such as Sweden, experienced a mild increase, and countries with a low baseline figure reported greater expansion of supported housing. Whether there will be a 'ceiling' effect preventing further increase once a threshold figure has been reached, remains to be seen.

Other factors that may also have contributed to the trend of "new institutionalization" in mental health care might include the difficulty of many patients to maintain independent lives in the community, the inability of community based services to provide sufficient support, underfunding of services in the community, family disintegration and a societal focus on individualism, hedonism and personal success with which mentally ill people may struggle to cope.

CONCLUSION

Reduction of psychiatric hospital beds has led to new forms of institutionalization beginning with supported housing, halfway houses and other forms of housing services in the community. Can it be concluded that the integration of most patients with severe mental illness into independent accommodation and regular employment has – if it ever existed – failed and that novel forms or institutionalization are required to care for a substantial number of these patients? In Israel, the Ministry of Health has established new specialized types of community facilities for older inpatients, and for younger patients without an institutional history (Grinshpoon et al., 2006).

This new institutionalization might be considered a social trend, in which the stigma associated with mental illness, and the public's ambivalence towards it, created the establishment of a new "psychiatric territory" in the community as compensation.

Fakhoury and Priebe (2007) also reported that despite the reduction of conventional psychiatric hospital beds in most Western industrialized countries, recent data suggest that we may already be witnessing a new phenomenon of 'reinstitutionalization'. There are remarkably similar trends in the provision of supported housing, the number of forensic beds and the increase in prison population in many countries. Though the number of psychiatric hospital beds decreased, changes in involuntary hospital admissions were inconsistent across countries. The question of whether the reduction of conventional hospital beds and the corresponding increase in supported housing and involuntary commitment should be described as reinstitutionalization or transinstitutionalization (suggesting a mere shifting of placements from one context to another) depends on the national balance between a further decrease in hospital beds on the one hand and newly established institutionalized care on the other. For example, in England, Spain and Sweden, the number of conventional psychiatric beds that were closed is greater than the total combined number of additional forensic beds and places in supported housing that were established during the same period. Though significant numbers of patients are now being cared for by multi-disciplinary teams in the community, others are probably part of the drastically increasing prison population. Thus, the total number of patients in institutional care might actually have increased. In Italy and The Netherlands the increase in forensic beds and supported housing has surpassed the decrease in conventional psychiatric bed numbers while Germany in there is more of a balance (Fakhoury and Priebe, 2007).

Priebe et al (2008) examined the factors that contributed to the increase in the provision of care in institutions and found a number of possible catalysts including: 1) greater morbidity, which may be associated with increased urbanization, altered lifestyles, and increased drug abuse; 2) growing opposition to risk that may result in increased referrals of patients to secure settings; 3) reduced informal support in the community for people with mental disorders; 4) a strong lobby of health care providers that led to increased funding for health care institutions.

There might also be a tendency among health care funders to transfer the financial responsibility of care for people with severe mental disorders to the social care sector, that often funds residential care and supervised and supported housing, or to the justice system, which funds prisons.

REFERENCES

Abramowitz M, Grinshpoon A, Priebe S, Ponizovsky AM. New institutionalization as a rebound phenomenon? The case of Israel. *Isr J Psychiatry Relat Sci* 2008;45:272-277.

Barbato A, D'Avanzo B, Rocca G, Amatulli A, Lampugnani D. A study of long-stay patients resettled in the community after closure of a psychiatric hospital in Italy. *Psychiatr Serv* 2004;55:67-70

Bauer A, Grinshpoon A, Rosca P, Khawaled R, Mester R, Yoffe R, Ponizovsky AM. Trends in involuntary psychiatric hospitalization in Israel 1991–2000. *Int J Law Psychiatry* 2007;30:60–70.

Central Bureau of Statistics. http://www.cbs.gov.il/reader/shnaton/templ_shnaton.html?num_tab=st06_11&CYear=2012 .

Clifford P, Charman A, Webb Y, Best S. Planning for community care. Long-stay populations of hospitals scheduled for rundown or closure. *Br J Psychiatry* 1991;158:190-196.

Desai MM, Rosenheck RA. Trends in discharge disposition, mortality, and service use among long-stay psychiatric patients in the 1990s. *Psychiatr Serv* 2003;54:542-548.

Fakhoury W, Priebe S. Deinstitutionalization and reinstitutionalization: major changes in the provision of mental healthcare. *Psychiatry* 2007;6:313-316.

Forchuk C, Joplin L, Schofield R, Csiernik R, Gorlick C, Turner K. Housing, income support and mental health: points of disconnection. *Health Res Policy Syst* 2007;12:5-14.

Grinshpoon A, Zilber N, Lerner Y, Ponizovsky A. Impact of rehabilitation legislation on the survival in the community of long-term patients discharged from psychiatric hospitals in Israel. *Soc Psychiatry Psychiatr Epidemiol* 2006;41:87–94.

Hamden A, Newton R, McCauley-Elsom K, Cross W. Is deinstitutionalization working in our community? *Int J Ment Health Nurs* 2011;20:274-283.

Holloway F. Community psychiatric care: from libertarianism to coercion. Moral panic and mental health policy in Britain. *Health Care Anal* 1996;4:235-243.

Hornik-Lurie T, Zilber N, Lerner Y. Trends in the use of rehabilitation services in the community by people with mental disabilities in Israel; the factors involved. *Isr J Health Policy Res* 2012;1:24.

Leff J, Trieman N, Gooch C. Team for the Assessment of Psychiatric Services (TAPS) Project 33: prospective follow-up study of long-stay patients discharged from two psychiatric hospitals. *Am J Psychiatry* 1996;153: 1318-1324.

Leff J, Trieman N. Long-stay patients discharged from psychiatric hospitals. *Br J Psychiatry* 2000;176:217-223.

Lelliott P, Wing J. A national audit of new long-stay psychiatric patients. II: Impact on services. *Br J Psychiatry* 1994;165:170-178.

Lichtenberg P, Kaplan Z, Grinshpoon A, Feldman D, Nahon D. The goals and limitations of Israel's psychiatric case register. *Psychiatr Serv* 1999;50: 1043-1048.

Machado V, Leonidas C, Santos MA, Souza J. Psychiatric readmission: an integrative review of the literature. *Int Nurs Rev* 2012;59:447-457.

Priebe S, Badesconyi A, Fioritti A, Hansson L, Kilian R, Torres-Gonzales F, Turner T, Wiersma D. Reinstitutionalisation in mental health care: comparison of data on service provision from six European countries. *BMJ* 2005;330:123-126.

Priebe S, Frottier P, Gaddini A, Kilian R, Lauber C, Martínez-Leal R, Munk-Jørgensen P, Walsh D, Wiersma D, Wright D. Mental health care institutions in nine European countries, 2002 to 2006. *Psychiatr Serv*2008;59:570-573.

Priebe S. Institutionalization revisited — with and without walls. *Acta Psychiatr Scand* 2004;110:81–82.

Rothbard AB, Kuno E, Schinnar AP, Hadley TR, Turk R.Service utilization and cost of community care for discharged state hospital patients: a 3-year follow-up study. *Am J Psychiatry* 1999;156:920-927.

Salize HJ, Dressing H. Epidemiology of involuntary placement of mentally ill people across the European Union. *Br J Psychiatry* 2004;184:163–168.

Scott J. Homelessness and mental illness. *Br J Psychiatry* 1993;162:314-324.

Thornicroft G, Gooch C, Dayson D. The TAPS project. 17: Readmission to hospital for long term psychiatric patients after discharge to the community. *BMJ* 1992;305:996-998.

Vázquez-Bourgon J, Salvador-Carulla L, Vázquez-Barquero JL. Community alternatives to acute inpatient care for severe psychiatric patients. *Actas Esp Psiquiatr* 2012;40:323-332.

Wall S, Hotopf M, Wessely S, Churchill R. Trends in the use of the Mental Health Act: England, 1984–96. *BMJ* 1999;318:1520–1521.

Weiser M, Kanyas K, Malaspina D, Harvey PD, Glick I, Goetz D, Karni O, Yakir A, Turetsky N, Fennig S, Nahon D, Lerer B, Davidson M. Sensitivity of ICD-10 diagnosis of psychotic disorders in the Israeli National Hospitalization Registry compared with RDC diagnoses based on SADS-L. *Compr Psychiatry* 2005;46:38-42.

Wing JK. How many psychiatric beds? *Psychol Med* 1971;1:188-190.

Chapter 6

MENTAL HEALTH LEGISLATION – CONSUMER'S PERSPECTIVE[*]

ABSTRACT

Mental health legislation and Information about involuntary psychiatric hospitalization (IPH) is crucial for the planning of national mental health care policy. In this chapter, the issues of IPH by court observation order and legal representation of involuntarily hospitalized patients and attitudes of personnel to this procedure are discussed, and illustrated with descriptions of actual court cases. Maximum security units and rehabilitative treatment settings for the forensic psychiatric inpatient population are described.

THE LAWS

The Law of Patient's Rights -1996 is a general law that governs the rights of all patients in the State of Israel. Because of the uniqueness and sensitivity of the treatment of patients with mental disorders, there is a specific Law for the Treatment of the Mentally Ill -1991 that governs the rights of individuals with mental disorders and defines the conditions under which a person can be admitted to a psychiatric hospital. The law replaced the Law for the Treatment of the Mentally Ill that was passed in -1955 (Khwaled and Grinshpoon, 2006).

---

[*] The chapter was written in collaboration with Razek Khwaled, R.N., M.A., L.Lb., Mental Health Services, Ministry of Health, Jerusalem, Israel

The aim of the Law for the Treatment of the Mentally Ill is to find a balance between the need to protect the public from people who are perceived as dangerous to themselves or to their environment owing to active symptoms of their illness, and to protect individuals who need treatment and who cope with active mental disorders. In addition, the Law for the Treatment of the Mentally Ill seeks to protect the basic freedoms and rights of individuals coping with psychiatric disorders. The appropriate balance between these goals is essentially achieved by defining the circumstances that allow for compulsory treatment and hospitalization, and by designation of procedures for supervision to prevent the abuse of the power granted to the authorities who implement the law.

In addition to these two laws, in the year 2000, the Law for the Rehabilitation of the Mentally Disabled in the Community, was passed, with the aim of providing for the rehabilitation and integration into the community of mentally disabled people, in order to allow them to achieve the highest possible level of functional independence and quality of life, while maintaining their dignity, in the spirit of the basic law: of human dignity and liberty. This law enables individuals with mental disorders to receive a rehabilitation basket appropriate to his/her needs in accord with the decisions of the Commission for Rehabilitation. The rehabilitation basket can include one or more domains listed in the law (supported housing, employment, leisure, education, etc.). In this chapter we will review a number of forensic psychiatry processes from the vantage point of the provision of care to patients while maintaining their basic rights.

PSYCHIATRIC HOSPITALIZATION

In Israel there are approximately 20,000 psychiatric hospitalizations per year, both voluntary and involuntary (Mental Health in Israel, 2012). Of them 5000 hospitalization are compulsory by order of the District Psychiatrist and 2000 by Court Order.

The issue of psychiatric hospitalization in general and involuntary hospitalization in particular and the trends throughout ten years, in Israel were examined (Bauer et al., 2007). In that analysis the authors found that the typical profile of the patient in involuntary hospitalization was a man, born in Israel, aged 18-24 or 65 years and older, living alone, with less than eight years of education, with a diagnosis of schizophrenia or delusional psychosis.

Table 1. Admissions to Psychiatric Hospitals and Legal Status

Year	Voluntary admissions	District Psychiatrist	Director	Court-ordered hospitalization	Court-ordered observation	Total
2007	15743	4134	119	356	1112	21464
2008	14756	4039	105	377	1221	20498
2009	14786	4199	94	363	1334	20776
2010	14938	4182	99	368	1321	20908
2011	14922	4493	131	391	1335	21272
2012	15098	4836	143	425	1655	22157

An additional study (Rosca et al., 2006), examined the characteristics of patients in a first involuntary admission to a psychiatric hospital, and identified a specific profile of patients with increased risk for future re-hospitalizations. The authors' hypothesis was that when the first hospital admission is involuntary, the number and duration of future hospitalizations would be greater.

The authors used information generated from the data base of psychiatric hospitalizations for all patients hospitalized for the first time in 1991 (n=2150), and a follow up of those patients throughout the next ten years. Chi-square statistics were used to examine significant differences in demographic variables between patients admitted voluntarily and those with involuntary hospital admissions. Multiple regression analysis was performed to identify a specific profile of risk for repeat hospitalization in the ten year period from 1991 to 2000.

Compared to patients admitted voluntarily, patients with involuntary admissions had significantly more and longer repeat hospitalizations and were more likely to be diagnosed with schizophrenia. Patients admitted voluntarily were more likely to be diagnosed with affective disorders. Risk factors for the number of repeat hospitalizations included: young age, legal status (involuntary) of first hospitalization, and duration of residence in Israel. Risk factors that impacted the duration of re-hospitalization were bachelorhood, widowhood, birthplace in Israel, and a suicide attempt prior to the first admission.

In accordance with the Law for the Treatment of the Mentally Ill, when there is prima facie evidence that a person has a mental disorder causing him/her to endanger him/herself or others, or if according to reports to the District Psychiatrists from a family physician, social worker or police, the District Psychiatrist is under the impression that there is basis for a psychiatric evaluation, he suggests that the individual be evaluated by a psychiatrist in either a public or private facility. In the absence of the patient's consent to be examined or to receive treatment, after contacting the District Psychiatrist, the District Psychiatrists may issue an order for a compulsory evaluation and based on the results decide if there is need for involuntary hospitalization.

DISTRICT PSYCHIATRIC COMMITTEE

Supervision of involuntary hospitalizations is the responsibility of the District Psychiatric Committee (Bauer et al., 2007), a statutory committee that decides whether or not to extend involuntary hospitalizations, rules on appeals, and decides on issues of compulsory hospitalization in criminal cases, such as granting leave, extension of confinement and discharge. Rulings of the District Psychiatric Committee can be appealed in the District Court.

Table 2. Trends in the number of cases brought before the District Psychiatric Committee

Year	Number of Cases
2007	6370
2008	8290
2009	8600
2010	8800
2011	9200
2012	10000

In order to protect the rights of individuals with mental disorders in compulsory hospitalization, or under court ordered hospitalization or an order for compulsory ambulatory care, in March 2004 the Law for the Treatment of the Mentally Ill 1991 was amended, (amendment no. 5, section 29) and now determines that every patient with mental disorders hospitalized involuntarily by either civil or criminal commitment, has the right for legal representation before the district psychiatric committee, at the expense of the State. The law determined that representation would begin gradual, and would be implemented in full in March 2007.

The authors examined the impact of the legal representation on the patient data of those who had representation by examining data from the current hospitalization and data from follow up across time (Bauer et al., 2008). Two patient groups with similar background data were compared. One group appeared before the District Psychiatric Committee with legal representation, and one group with no representation. Findings revealed significant between group differences.

Higher percentages of patients that had legal representation returned both to involuntary and voluntary hospitalization than patients that had no representation. In addition, duration of time after discharge until re-hospitalization was shorter among patients that had representation, and the duration of hospitalization was longer than for patients without legal representation.

These results that are most significant have one possible explanation, and that is that the attorney represents the wishes of the patient, rather that his/her welfare. In order to achieve his/her goal, the attorney uses all possible legal arguments to discharge patients and the patients are then discharged prematurely, before completing their treatment. The physicians argue that treatment can be completed even if the patients do not meet the conditions prescribed by the law and that the law should be viewed in a broader perspective.

To distinguish from the first group that had legal representation, the second group, and the patients that appeared before the Psychiatric Committee were not aware of the nuances of the legal arguments. Similarly, the authors examined the attitudes of medical professionals concerning the issue of legal representation. Grinshpoon et al (2011) conducted a study that included hospital staff members who completed a designated research questionnaire at two time points: one month before and one year following the implementation of the legal representation. Participants included 37 registered psychiatric nurses, 18 psychiatrists and 12 psychiatric social workers. There was a 74% response rate for the entire study sample, 98% nurses, 65% for the other professionals. In the beginning of the study, 64% of the responders (43 out of 67) confirmed positive attitude items and 55% (37 out of 67) confirmed negative attitude items on the scale (Table 3).

Abramowitz et al (2011) performed a survey comparing the attitudes of medical students and law students concerning legal representation of individuals with mental disorders. No significant between-group differences were found regarding the general attitude towards people with mental disorders, and the positive position regarding legal representation.

Table 3. Changes in attitudes of mental health professionals regarding legal representation

Hospital staff group	Before legal representation introduced (N=67)		One year after legal representation introduced (N=67)		Paired t-test	
	Mean	SD	Mean	SD	t-value	p
Psychiatric nurses (n=37)						
Positive attitudes	2.44	0.38	2.35	0.47	0.87	0.38
Negative attitudes	2.71	0.54	2.40	0.57	2.56	0.015
Other professionals (n=30)						
Positive attitudes	2.46	0.50	2.15	0.48	0.45	0.65
Negative attitudes	3.00	0.38	3.01	0.48	0.02	0.98
Total sample (n=67)						
Positive attitudes	2.41	0.45	2.33	0.48	0.88	0.38
Negative attitudes	2.86	0.55	2.66	0.57	2.51	0.015
ANOVA with Tukey post-hoc single comparisons						
Positive attitudes	F_3=6.87, p<.001		--	--	--	--
Negative attitudes	F_3 =5.28, p=.03		--	--	--	--

PSYCHIATRY AND LEGAL PROCEEDINGS

I. The Specialist in Forensic Psychiatry is a Physician Whose Primary Specialty is Psychiatry

The forensic psychiatrist is called upon to provide an expert professional opinion, evaluation and appropriate treatment for individuals who stand trial, after breaking the law, when the judge and the attorneys need to know, in accord with the law, whether the individual is sane, or whether his thoughts, opinions and behavior result from insanity, or a mental disorder.

In all cases where the judge or attorneys argue that the mental state of the accused is in doubt, according to various laws of the legal system, it must be proven by a psychiatric specialist in court. The forensic psychiatrist's professional evaluations often determine the legal verdict and the sentence, whether or not the accused will sit in prison or in a psychiatric hospital to received appropriate treatment for his mental disorder.

The forensic psychiatrist's expert opinion is generally required in broad areas of the legal system. In criminal law that deals with murder, rape, abuse and so forth, the role of the forensic psychiatrist in most cases is to express his opinion, whether or not the accused can stand trial and an additional question is whether the defendant was sane or mentally insane at the time of the criminal act. The decision of the judge ruling in this type of criminal law sends the defendant to an ambulatory psychiatric evaluation, or for inpatient psychiatric observation, after which the physician with the assistance of other staff members prepares an expert opinion for the Court that relates to the question of insanity at the time of the crime, and the question of the capacity to stand trial (Grinshpoon et al., 2011) found that 83% of the people sent for observation do not receive a psychiatric diagnosis, and are returned to the legal system. However a 10-year follow-up of these individuals revealed that 56% of them were ultimately given a psychiatric diagnosis (Figure 1).

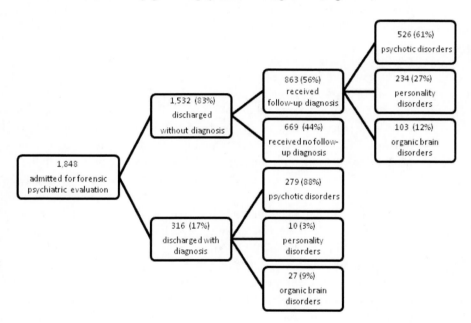

Figure 1. Observation orders and psychiatric diagnoses (reprinted with permission from Gninshpoon et al., 2011).

The data presented above show a steady rise in the number of court orders for psychiatric observation. The following solutions are recommended for dealing with the increasing amount of orders and for the expansion of the interface between the legal and psychiatric systems:

A. Court liaison and diversion scheme – Forensic psychiatric consulting services in the court, and routing schemes. The goal is to remove individuals with mental disorders from the legal system, and to refer them to appropriate mental health facilities for treatment, as soon as possible. A range of professional, therapeutic, economic and humanitarian considerations led to the development of psychiatric consultations in prisons and in the courts, as early as the beginning of the twentieth century in the United States. Therapeutic entities near the courts provided information to the court and recommended appropriate treatment facilities for the patients. The clinic had a multidisciplinary staff with a psychiatrist, an assistant psychiatrist, nurses, and a secretary. In addition to the examination of the patient, emphasis was placed on collecting all relevant medical information about the patient. By the end of the 1980's, hundreds of clinics were established in the United States of America, most of which were in the vicinity of high level courts, and whose primary purpose was to make a comprehensive psychiatric evaluation available to the court, without hospitalization. In England and Wales similar consulting services of vital assistance to the courts were established at the end of the nineties. The psychiatric consultation teams are located in the Magistrate's Court and also provide services to regional police stations. The teams were established to raise awareness of mental illness in the courts, and the role focused on the evaluation of detainees. When indeed mental disorders were diagnosed, patients were referred for treatment in an appropriate mental health facility, using involuntary hospitalization, civil or criminal commitment (Vaughan, 2003)

   The efficacy of the process was examined in a number of cases and it was clear that as a result of the activities of the multi-disciplinary teams there was an increase in the identification of psychiatric morbidity in the jails, and there was then a reduction in the time lapse from arrest to hospitalization. By the end of the 1990's, In England and Wales there were 150 such services, however owing to lack of funding and manpower, their number declined. In 2005 there was renewed interest in the British government to revive the services (James, 2006). Similar services were established in Australia and in New Zealand.

B. Mental Health Courts - Specialized courts. The courts are affected by social changes and are in the forefront of coping with a spectrum of problems such as drug use, domestic violence and mental illness. Mental Health Courts were established in the United States in the mid 1990's. These courts were established to cope with the growing number of prisoners in the jails who were diagnosed with mental disorders and in response to the complicated dilemmas that faced the courts in those cases (Watson et al., 2001), and to prevent criminality or repeat offenses among the mentally ill. The court officials, including the judge, the prosecutor and the defense attorneys have specialized training in psychiatry and are familiar with the local psychiatric systems. The efficient operation of the designated courts was examined in several studies that demonstrated a decline in the rates of repeat offenses and new violent crimes (Mcniel and Binder 2007; Trupin and Richards, 2003).

II. Prolonged Court Ordered Commitment

Criminal appeal 3854/02 v. District Psychiatric Committee ruled on the issue of prolonged court ordered hospitalization. Mr. A was prosecuted for criminal charges of assault and theft. District court determined based on the expert opinion of the District Psychiatrist that A suffered from a mental disorder and did not have the capacity to stand trial. The Court ordered, in accord with the Law for the Treatment of the Mentally Ill, involuntary hospitalization for A. While hospitalized the patient was served with an additional indictment for an injurious attack and threats to his mother. Court ordered hospitalization was issued for this second indictment. A approached the District Psychiatric committee and asked to cancel the court order and to discharge him. In this request he argued that the physicians in the department where he was hospitalized determined that he was not at risk for suicide or for violence toward others, and that he was eligible for vacations. The District Psychiatric Committee rejected his request to be discharged. The committee determined that he was at a high risk for danger to himself and to others. However, the Committee decided to approve short vacations. A appealed arguing that there was no justification for issuing a court ordered hospitalization that was not time limited, and argued that there was no reason to challenge, certainly without explanation - the decisions of the attending physicians. The District Court ruled in the appeal that the court order was not time limited. In addition, the court ruled that the Psychiatric Committee was authorized to determine, based on its experience that A was a danger to himself and to others. In addition, the court ordered the Committee to re-examine A's condition within one month to consider whether he was fit to be discharged or alternatively to decide on additional mitigating measures in the event that he no longer posed an actual threat. In accord with the court's ruling the committee discussed the case again and determined that A would not be released from involuntary hospitalization because he was still dangerous. However, the duration of his vacations was extended. A appealed the ruling of the District Court to the Supreme Court, and argued that the court ordered hospitalization with no time limit, in criminal proceedings, was unreasonable and disproportionate.

Following this ruling a number of serious issues were raised including:

A. There is no overlap or connection between the duration of hospitalization and duration of incarceration for the crime committed. In other words, a person who is not mentally ill and is tried for a petty offense may receive a relatively short prison sentence, in comparison to a person with mental illness who committed the same crime and was sent for a prolonged court-ordered hospitalization. This is a complicated situation. Some claim that it is not just, ethical or reasonable that a person remain for a long period of time in involuntary court ordered hospitalization where the conditions of hospitalization in legal terms are stricter than those under civil commitment, and certainly in comparison to voluntary hospitalization. For example, the issue of vacations – in court ordered hospitalization, the District Psychiatric Committee must approve vacations, and that is not required for civil commitment or for voluntary hospitalizations where vacations are determined at the discretion of the attending physician with no intervention by the District Psychiatric Committee. The President of the Supreme Court at that time, the Honorable Judge Barak, ruled that the legislature must settle the matter, and indeed a bill was introduced, which has not yet been accepted, according to which a court that orders psychiatric hospitalization will determine the maximum length of hospitalization that does not exceed the length of time a person would have been sent to jail. Until legislation is passed, the Honorable Judge Barak recommended changing involuntary hospitalization from the "criminal track", e.g., court ordered hospitalization, to the "civilian track", e.g., civil confinement.

B. In contrast to the case described in the above verdict, there could be a potential situation where the patient that committed a serious crime (such as murder) is sent to court ordered hospitalization. The patient is sent to the hospital for treatment and not for incarceration because the court proved that the patient did not bear criminal responsibility owing to his mental disorders. In that case, the patient might be discharged after a relatively short period if his mental state improved and if there is no medical justification for continuing involuntary hospitalization in a psychiatric hospital. The problem: there are those who argue that discharging patients, who committed serious crimes, even if they are currently in remission, might endanger the public because it is likely that for at least some of the patients there is a tendency for violent behavior. The dangerousness of those patients might increase because in some cases it is not possible to conduct regular follow up in the community, and they then do not receive all of the medication necessary to restrain their aggression. This is especially relevant when dealing with a patient that is not in a supportive environment or a patient with low compliance to treatment.

Following the above ruling two steps were taken:

- A bill was drawn, regarding the duration of hospitalization of a person with court ordered hospitalization, according to which the length of the court ordered hospitalization should be for a period of time not exceeding the period of time that the criminal proceedings would continue if the person was convicted for the crime for which he was being tried.
- Bauer et al (2005) performed a survey in the forensic psychiatry department of the Department of Mental Health. They collected data about patients under court ordered psychiatric hospitalizations for periods of ten years or more, and found that at that time there were 65 patients under court ordered hospitalization for longer than ten years. The authors approached the hospitals in accord with the court ruling, to see if according to the condition of the patients the involuntary court ordered hospitalizations could be changed to voluntary hospitalizations or civil commitments or even discharge of the patients.

III. The Penal Code is the Primary Law That Defines the Various Criminal Offenses

The expected sentence for each criminal offense is defined in the law. The sentence is the maximum penalty that can be imposed on a person convicted for the same offence, and the court may impose any penalty that does not exceed the penalty prescribed by the law for that offense.

The exception to the rule is murder. The sentence for a person convicted of murder is life imprisonment. The court has no discretion and must sentence a person convicted of murder with life imprisonment. This strict rule often creates difficulties because there are cases, when despite the gravity of the offense of murder, it seems inappropriate to ignore unique circumstances of a case, and impose life imprisonment.

Throughout the years there were a number of cases that caused legislators to conclude that even when the offense is murder, special cases should be left to the discretion of the court and should allow the court to deviate from the mandatory life sentence and to impose a penalty on those convicted of murder based on the discretion of the court given the unique circumstances of the case.

Thus, the penal code was amended in 1995, and Clause 300A that determines a reduced sentence for a person convicted of murder under the enumerated circumstances, such that life imprisonment is not mandatory and the court is authorized to give a lighter sentence taking into account the circumstances of the case.

The circumstances that allow for reduced sentences are:

1. The defendant was in a state that owing to a severe mental disorder or impairment in mental capacity had a substantially limited capacity to understand what he was doing, or to refrain from committing the act but not to the point of absolute exemption from liability, as determined in the insanity defense.
2. The defendant is in a state where his actions somewhat exceeded the reasonable boundaries required for self-defense, need or necessity.

The defendant was in a state of severe emotional distress / following severe prolonged abuse either by a family member, or by the person whose death the defendant caused.

The first case where a reduced sentence was given for murder was the case of a defendant who murdered a British tourist and harmed the tourist's companion. The court sentenced the defendant to 20 years for both crimes (murder and severe injury with intent) after determining that the defendant suffered from a severe mental disorder, though it was not a mental disorder that relieves the defendant of criminal responsibility.

After the amendment was passed, a committee was established by the Israel Psychiatric Association, to formulate a position paper regarding the amendment and to provide guidelines for psychiatrists that are called to give expert psychiatric opinions during which the question of reduced punishment might arise.

Forensic psychiatry is also required in civil law that deals with mental impairment (in order to determine social security payments for mental impairment), to approve wills, to determine guardianship and so forth. With the aid of a forensic psychiatrist's expert opinion, the judge is able to rule, in cases the majority of which will considerably impact the life of the person on trial or the lives of his family members.

For example: a psychiatric expert opinion for a person who changed his will or for a person who is ill and can no long care for himself or his property and requires a guardian to make various decisions for him/her while he/she is still alive.

EVALUATION OF DANGEROUSNESS

Mental health caregivers across the world use the Historical, Clinical Risk Management – 20 scale to evaluate dangerousness among individuals with mental impairments.

The instruments allows weighting of 20 parameters related to the individual's personal history (past violence, substance abuse, mental disorders) to current clinical findings (impulsivity, negative attitudes, non-compliance with treatment) and future risk factors (such as refusal to take medication or to participate in therapy, pressure) to a numeric index that reflects the probability of future violence (low, medium or high probability).

In order to use the instrument in Israel, a survey of risk assessment instruments for use among the mentally ill was performed (Bauer, 2002), after which the Department of Mental Health Services in the Ministry of Health initiated a study to validate a Hebrew version of the HCL-20, in three mental health centers, Sha'ar Menashe, Lev Hasharon and the mental health services of the prison authority. After a two year study, the Hebrew version of the instrument was validated and will soon be implemented in the routine assessment of dangerousness among patients, when necessary, and especially at the beginning of involuntary hospitalization and when making decisions to extend it (Ivgi et al., 2014).

ADAPTING THE TREATMENT SETTING TO THE PATIENT POPULATION

People who suffer from mental disorders are on a broad spectrum and need settings appropriate to their conditions, special needs. The Ministry of Health strives to advance and develop settings to provide optimal care for the patient populations with special needs. The settings include:

The Maximum Security Unit at Sha'ar Menashe Mental Health Center

In 1997 a maximum security unit was established. The unit includes four departments of 32 beds each, with a total of 128 beds. The unit is a national facility that includes rehabilitation. The center treats patients under court ordered hospitalization, and especially violent patients. The unit has developed unique methods for dealing with violent patients and for providing multi-disciplinary expert opinions that include psychiatric, psychological and criminological aspects. The inpatients in the unit are treated until they achieve balanced mental states, after which they are transferred to the rehabilitation department (72 beds) in preparation for discharge.

In 1999 the Director of Mental Health Services in the Israel Ministry of Health established a committee that drafted Rules and Regulations for operation of the Maximum Security Unit, including guidelines for referral and a definition of violent behavior. The following rules were adopted for referral of patients to the National Maximum Security Unit:

- Mental disorder
- Age 18-65
- Involuntary hospitalization
- The patient is a danger to his/her environment following high levels of aggression toward others that cannot be restrained in a standard closed ward, and for those who committed murder or serious assault and managed to escape other inpatient settings.

A Unique Rehabilitation Department in Sha'ar Menashe Mental Health Center

The department is designed to treat a range of serious psychopathologies, with various treatment interventions for closed inpatient populations in the hospital and for patients from the maximum security unit, who are scheduled for discharge in partial or complete remission. The rehabilitation department helps them acquire the skills necessary for integration into the general community.

The target population includes patients with severe schizophrenia who performed crimes while in active psychotic states mainly related to schizophrenia and associated morbidities of personality disorders or psycho-active substance abuse. In the rehabilitation department emphasis is on promoting the rehabilitation process, development of skills for independent functioning, learning Hebrew and English, becoming acquainted with community based rehabilitation services and participating in local leisure time activities. There is a wide range of social and leisure time activities in the rehabilitation department such as participation in clubhouse activities in the hospital and community based clubhouse activities for younger and older persons coping with mental disorders. In the afternoons the social activities in the clubhouse include board games, watching movies, computer activities, in a relaxed and fun-filled atmosphere. Rehabilitation patients take an active role in hospital events such as sports competitions with patients from other hospitals, and social events in honor of holidays, and other special events. The theme of the rehabilitation department is "a healthy mind in a healthy body" and it promotes awareness of physical activity, sports, and health eating. To promote adjustment outside the hospital, a classroom project for further education of the inpatients in planned for all patients in the ward.

Therapeutic Residence and Intensive Therapeutic Residence

These residences are designed for patients with chronic mental disorders for whom the standard housing facilities for community based rehabilitation are not suitable, though rehabilitation might be a viable option in the future. In the therapeutic residence patients are accompanied and assisted in all facets of daily living and receive medical, employment and social support. There are currently 540 beds for patients with different levels of severity of illness, including patients with physical illnesses in addition to their mental disorders.

Staff Training Programs for Treatment of Drugs as Addictions at Psychiatric Hospitals and Designated Beds for the Treatment of This Patient Population

Target population: psychiatrists, nursing staff, social workers, psychologists, clinical criminologists, para-medical employees.

Rationale: The term dual diagnosis describes the use of psycho-active substances alongside a psychiatric disorder. Research has shown that 30% - 60% of psychiatric patients have a dual diagnosis. This population has unique characteristics, diagnostic and treatment methods. In practice, there are patients that "fall between the chairs" and do not received appropriate clinical and rehabilitation therapy, and who are referred to various other services.

The Knesset (Israeli Parliament) committee that discussed the fight against drugs, decided to train medical personnel and para-medical staff members in this field and in the treatment of these patients because they realized that dual diagnosis patients make up a major share of all patients with mental disorders. In addition, in the near future more beds in psychiatric hospitals will be designated for dual diagnosis patients.

In order to make the subject accessible to caregivers that came from various medical and paramedical disciplines, and to enable them to acquire the tools to treat dual diagnosis patients a training program based on state of the art knowledge of dual diagnosis was compiled, to offer services, treatment and rehabilitation tailored to the unique needs of that population. Five hundred multi-disciplinary caregivers in the field of mental health, from all psychiatric hospitals participated in the training programs. In addition to the existing dual diagnosis departments there are now a number of designated dual diagnosis beds in additional hospitals.

Planning Treatment Settings for Special Needs Populations

The Ministry of Health and the Ministry of Welfare have recently had joint discussions to finalize the nature, rules and regulations for the settings designed for the treatment of individuals with psychiatric symptoms in addition to severe cognitive impairment, head injuries, and a history of physical illnesses. This population requires attention tailored to the unique needs both in terms of treatment and physical space necessary for optimal care.

Therapeutic Residential Rehabilitation Settings

Recently, rehabilitation settings have been established for individuals coping with mental disorders who do not require hospitalization, but are not yet ready for sheltered housing facilities in the community. The settings are designed for individuals who need guidance and assistance in all facets of daily life, and will enable optimal quality of life for the residents. There are plans for 200 beds in the rehabilitation facilities. According to the estimates, 74% of the residents will be transferred from other rehabilitation settings such as treatment facilities, long-term hospitalization and rehabilitation hostels.

Mental Health Reform

The National Health Insurance Law passed in 1994 includes three key measures:

- Regulation of the rights of residents and citizens to receive health care
- Definition of basket of health services

Transfer of Most Health Services to the Health Funds

When the law was legislated, mental health services, geriatric medicine, and preventive medicines were not included in the basket of services under the responsibility of the health funds.

Throughout the years, there was discussion regarding three reforms in mental health care: structural, rehabilitation, and those related to insurance. The structural reform relates mainly to the reduction of the number of psychiatric inpatient beds from 7000 in the 1990's to 3000 inpatient beds today. The component of rehabilitation in the reform relates mainly to the rehabilitation settings in the community that were established after the legislation of the Law for the Rehabilitation of the Mentally Ill in the Community, in 2000, and the increase in the number of rehabilitees from 1000 to 20,000.

The goal of the insurance reform in mental health is to transfer the responsibility for provision of mental health care from the Ministry of Health to the health funds (Elisha and Grinshpoon, 2007), within the framework of the National Health Insurance Law. This change will enable people with mental disorders to receive both inpatient and ambulatory care from their health funds, just like any other person that suffers from a medical condition, and without discrimination or stigma.

Since the enactment of the National Health Insurance Law, the Ministry of Health has worked with the health funds and the Ministry of Finance to transfer mental health care to the funds. According to this program, the responsibility for mental health care will be transferred to the health funds in accordance with the National Health Insurance order 2012, issued by the Minister of Health pursuant to his authority under the National Health Insurance law.

The program was approved by the cabinet, and was granted status of a government decision and will come into effect in the beginning of July 2015. Until that time, the Ministry of Health will continue to provide mental health services and will prepare to transfer responsibility to the health funds a according to schedule.

Following the reform, the budget for mental health care in the community will be doubled, as will the number of recipients of care in the community clinics. These applicants for care are currently treated in expensive private settings, or wait extended periods of time for an appointment for treatment.

REFERENCES

Abramowitz M, Bentov-Gofrit B, Khawaled R, Bauer A, Cohen TI. Attitudes among medical and law students toward decision-making in regard to involuntary psychiatric hospitalization. *Int J Law Psychiatry* 2011;34: 368–373.

Bauer A , Gruszniewsky A , Khawaled R, Grinshpoon A , Mark M, Mester R. Reflections on dangerousness and its prediction — a truly tantalizing task. *Med Law* 2002;21:495-520.

Bauer A, Rosca P, Grinshpoon A, Khawalled R, Mester R. Regional psychiatric boards in Israel: expectations and   realities. *Int J Law Psychiatry* 2005;28:661-669.

Bauer A, Rusca P, Grinshpoon A, Khawalled R, Mester R. Monitoring long-term court order psychiatric hospitalization: a pilot project in Israel. *J Med Law* 2006;25:83-99

Bauer A, Rosca P , Grinshpoon A, Khawalled R, Mester R, Yoffe R, Ponizovsky AM. Trends in involuntary psychiatric hospitalization in Israel 1991-2000 *Int J Law Psychiatry* 2007;30:60-70.

Bauer A, Khawaled R, Rosca P, Ponizovsky AM. Legal representation is associated with psychiatric readmissions. *Open Law J* 2008;1:6-10.

Elisha D, Grinshpoon A. Mental health reform in Israel: how to increase the opportunities and reduce the threats Harefuah 2007;146:291-296 (in Hebrew).

Grinshpoon A, Khawaled R, Levy T, Rosca P, Ponizovsky AM. Changes in psychiatric nurse attitudes towards legal representation of inpatients at district psychiatric board hearings in Israel: a pilot study. *Open J Psychiatry*, 2011;1:126-131.

Grinshpoon A, Khawaled R, Polakiewicz J, Appelbaum PS, Ponizovsky AM. Psychiatric hospitalization by court observation order in Israel: A ten-year follow-up study. *Isr J Psychiatry Relat Sci* 2011;48:201-206.

James DV. Court diversion in perspective. *Aust NZ J Psychiatry* 2006;40:529-538.

Ivgi D, Bauer A, Khawaled R, Rosca P, Weiss Y, Ponizovsly AM. Validation of the HCR-20 scale for assessment risk of violent behavior in Israeli psychiatric inpatients. *Isr J Psychiatry Relat Sci* 2014 (in press).

Khwaled R, Grinshpoon A. Israel's Mental Health Treatment Act: Amendments past and future. *Med Law* 2006;35:100-112.

McNiel DE, Binder RL. Effectiveness of a mental health court in reducing criminal recidivism and violence. *Am J Psychiatry* 2007;164:1395-1403.

Mental Health in Israel. Statistical Annual 2012. Ministry of Health, Jerusalem, 2012.

Rosca P, Bauer A, Grinshpoon A, Khawaled R, Mester R, Ponizovsky AM. Rehospitalizations among psychiatric patients whose first admission was involuntary: A 10-year follow-up. *Isr J Psychiatry Relat Sci* 2006;43:57-64.

Trupin E, Richards H. Seattle's mental health courts: early indicators of effectiveness. *Int J Law Psychiatry* 2003;26:33-53.

Vaughan P, Austen C, Le Feuvre M, O'Grady J, Swyer B. Psychiatric support to magistrates' courts. *Med Sci Law* 2003;43:255-259.

Watson A, Hanrahan P, Luchins D, Lurigio A. Mental health courts and the complex issue of mentally ill offenders. *Psychiatr Serv* 2001;52:477-481.

Chapter 7

NEED FOR MENTAL HEALTH SERVICES AND TREATMENT LAG[*]

ABSTRACT

In previous chapters we described need for psychiatric services among patients diagnosed with SMI and mental health services' responses to these demands. In the current chapter we discuss our investigations of patients who sought professional psychiatric help for psychological symptoms and therefore attended outpatient clinics for the first time in their lives. Describing our findings, we will focus on ethnic differences between Israeli Arabs and Jews in help-seeking behavior, psychiatric diagnosis detection, and experienced emotional distress and psychosocial resources.

Although studies indicate that the early recognition and timely treatment of common psychiatric disorders helps reduce suffering, prevents mental disabilities and makes interventions more cost-effective (Ho and Andreasen, 2001; Ho et al., 2003), there is often a considerable time lag between the onset of psychiatric disorder and help-seeking (Amaddeo et al., 2001; Wang et al., 2002; Bijl et al., 2003; Kohn et al., 2004) and many people do not seek professional help at all (Andrews et al., 2001; Laukkala et al., 2001; Oliver et al., 2005). The adverse effects of treatment delay have been well documented: people who leave a disorder untreated tend to have a poorer outcome in the

[*] This chapter is based on two articles that were published in the Israel Journal of Psychiatry (Ponizovsky et al., 2007 a, b), sections of which are reproduced here with the permission of the Editor in Chief).

short- and long-term (Loebel et al., 1992; Carbone et al., 1999; Larsen et al., 2000; Melle et al., 2004).

A number of illness-related characteristics, as well as socio-cultural factors, have been identified as contributing to treatment delay: young age at onset of the disorder (Kessler et al., 1998; Wang et al., 2004); insidious onset (Larsen et al., 1996); negative symptoms (Draje et al., 2000); low social class (Mulvany et al., 2001); the attitudes and belief systems prevalent in a society, including the stigmatization of mental illness (Angermeyer et al., 1999; Sirey 2001; Lauber et al., 2006) and poor psychosocial support (Drake et al., 2000; Larsen et al., 1998; Barnes et al., 2000).

Only a few psychiatric epidemiological studies in Arab countries and published in English have included measures of psychological distress (Ghubash et al., 1992; Ghubash et al., 2001; Abou-Saleh et al., 2001). Some of those studies included a calibration of the scale used as a screening instrument in a two-stage diagnostic procedure (Abou-Saleh et al., 2001). Other studies used the measures solely as an indicator of psychological distress and a proxy for psychopathology (Abdel-Khalek, 1998; Becker et al., 2002).

In Israel two studies on psychological distress have been published on the Arab minority: one on the elderly living in the community (Shemesh et al., 2006) and a more recent survey on adults aged 21 and above, which was part of the World Health Survey (Levav et al., 2007). Both studies used the GHQ-12 (Goldberg and Williams, 1988) to detect distress. In both studies the scores were considerably higher among Israeli Arabs than among the Jews, even with suitable controls entered into the analysis. However, when an ad hoc measure of suspected psychopathology was introduced, a multivariate analysis found no difference in the scores (Shemesh et al., 2006). In contrast, Levav et al (2007) found that Israeli Arabs had higher GHQ-12 mean scores and lower self-assessed mental health when compared to Jewish-Israelis. Arab subjects declared their intention to seek specialized health care only when high distress scores accompanied their depression and anxiety disorders. The question then arises as to whether questionnaire response style is responsible for the difference between the two population groups and that the score disparities are not a "true" reflection of mental status.

Two illustrations from two different contexts support the case for studying this issue. In the United States, a study of 98 elderly Muslim immigrants found that the respondents were likely to report their mental health and life satisfaction to be poorer than the interviewers perceived (Salari, 2002). In Al-Ain in the United Arab Emirates, a study reported that the SRQ-based "caseness" was eight times higher than the ICD-10 diagnosis, based on the

Composite International Diagnostic Interview (Robbins et al., 2088). This suggests a possible tendency to complain or, alternatively, to agree with questionnaire items, particularly when answers are dichotomized ("yes sayers") (Abyad, 2001).

Israel, a multi-ethnic society with an extensive network of public psychiatric settings (Levav and Grinshpoon, 2004), provides a suitable context for investigating the relationship between cultural variables attributable to ethnic affiliation and the expression of psychological distress in outpatients, and a suitable ground for investigating the relationship between delay in treatment-seeking and cultural barriers to health care. Obviously, most or all of these patients defined their psychopathology as requiring psychiatric care, and most or all had overcome the barriers raised by stigma to seeking the help of a psychiatric clinic. The fact that both population groups (Arabs and Jews) are voluntary outpatients, rather than a heterogeneous sample living in the community, makes them, we are entitled to assume, comparable. The findings of such a study should leave mental health policy makers, care providers, and users and their families better informed for program planning.

The study reported here is a part of survey on treatment lag among first-time adult psychiatric outpatients. The study objective was to compare the level of expression of psychological distress between Israeli Arabs and Jews, while controlling for confounding factors, e.g., sociodemographic variables. Clinician's diagnoses and self-reported mental health problems were registered as clinical outcome variables and measures of self-efficacy and perceived social support as personal psychosocial resources. The rationale for selecting these variables was as follows: 1) socio-demographic factors, such as gender (Denton et al., 2004; Grzywacz et al., 2004) and education (Grzywacz et al., 2004; Shields, 2004), have been shown repeatedly to be associated with emotional distress scores; 2) social support acts as a buffer against the effects of an adverse environment (Kessler et al., 1985; Turner and Marino, 1994; Norris and Kaniasty, 1996; Olstad et al., 2001; Regehr and Hemsworth, 2001; Kornblith et al., 2001) while encouraging adaptability (Thoits, 1995); and 3) self-efficacy is a measure of belief in one's ability to negotiate stressful situations (Schwarzer, 2002; Fry and Debats, 2002; Wu et al., 2004).

METHODS

Study Design

At the center of the study was the first-ever visit by an adult to a psychiatric clinic. In the pilot stage we tested the reliability of 20 patients' self-report with regard to the onset of the current disorder against the information obtained at intake by a qualified clinician. The questionnaire used in this study was translated from Hebrew into Arabic and Russian, to match the patient's language of preference. The self-report questionnaire was administered to all consecutive clinic patients making a first-time visit between December 2001 and November 2002.

The Clinics

Three psychiatric clinics participated. They were chosen from Israel's main geographical regions: north and south Galilee, including both urban and rural centers, and the central Dan region, with both urban and suburban population centers, including inner city and immigrant groups. The clinics were located in a psychiatric hospital, in a general hospital, and in a freestanding outpatient clinic. In the outpatient clinic serving predominantly Arab patients, the psychiatrist participated in the study was Arab by origin, while in other two clinics the specialists were Jewish origin. The Institutional Review Board for Human Studies approved the study protocol in each clinic.

The Sample

Of a total of 354 apparently first-time attendees, only 251 fulfilled the inclusion criteria, 1) they were seeking help from a psychiatrist for mental health problems for the first time in their life, and 2) they gave written informed consent to their participation in the study. Of the 103 patients not enrolled, 87 were not in fact first-time attendees and 16 refused to be interviewed. The latter did not differ from the participants by age and gender distribution. The sample was divided by ethnic origin into an Arab (n=75) and a Jewish (n=176) sub-sample. The former subgroup comprised of 98% Muslim Arabs and the latter included only 4% Russian-born Jewish immigrants. All comparisons were performed between these two subgroups.

Procedure

During the intake interview, and once informed consent had been given, all patients aged 21-65 seeking care for any mental health problem answered a questionnaire that took 25 minutes to complete. The intake clinician made a psychiatric diagnosis on ICD-10 criteria, which was recorded on a separate form. To assure confidentiality, the clinician erased the patient's name from both coded forms. A separate notebook kept by the clinic investigator recorded both the patient's name and code for any future reference.

The Instruments

A *36-item questionnaire* included items on the time elapsed between the onset of the presenting symptom(s) and the current clinic visit; source of referral; reasons for the treatment lag; main complaints of mental health; current psychiatric problems (self-diagnosis); attitudes to psychiatric disorders and treatment; pathways to care; and standard socio-demographic information.

Socio-Demographic Questionnaire
The questionnaire consisted of (a) a section on socio-demographic information (gender, age, marital status, years of schooling, employment, and religious observance).

The General Health Questionnaire
In particular its abridged 12-item version (GHQ-12) has been used extensively world-wide (Usturi and Sartorius, 1993), including Israel and Arab countries (Abou-Saleh et al., 2001). It is a valid and reliable measure of current non-specific psychological distress (Goldberg and Williams, 2002; Dohrenwend et al., 1980). The scale asks whether the respondent has experienced a particular symptom or behavior within the last month. The subjects answer questions, on a 4-point scale, ranging from "much less than usuall" (score 0) to "much more than usual" (score 3). In accordance with past research, items scored two or three were regarded as positive and given a score of one. Ratings were summarized across the 12 items to give an individual GHQ score ranging between 0 and 12. Following current practice, an overall score of three or higher was regarded as indicative of a "case" of emotional distress (May, 1992; Piccinelli et al., 1993).

The General Self-Efficacy Scale (GSES)

The GSES measures belief in one's ability to cope with stressful situations (Schwarzer and Jerusalem, 2002). The scale consists of 10 items (e.g., "Usually I am able to control a situation" or "In unexpected situations, I always know how I must behave myself"). Responses are rated on a 4- point Likert-scale ranging from "absolutely not true" (weighted as 1) to "absolutely true" (weighted as 4), where the higher GSES total scores indicate stronger confidence in self-efficacy. Good internal reliability consistency (*alpha* = .92) and test-retest reliability over six months have been reported (Cheung and Sun, 1999; Skaret et al., 2003). This scale has been applied to physicians and nurses in primary care in Israel (Rabin et al., 2000; Idel et al., 2003) as well as to psychiatric inpatients (Ritsner et al., 2000).

The Multidimensional Scale of Perceived Social Support (MSPSS) (Zimet et al., 1988)

Is a self-report instrument for assessment of emotional help and the level of satisfaction with social support obtained from three sources - family, friends and significant others. The scale comprises 12 items, which refer to people to whom the respondent would turn if he/she had problems in the past month of a personal, health or family nature, as well as financial and employment problems (e.g., "I get the emotional help and support I need from my family", or "I have friends with whom I can share my joys and sorrows", or "There is a special person who is around when I am in need"). Responses are scored on a 7-point scale from 1 ('completely disagree') to 7 ('completely agree'). An MSPSS index and three subscales – family, friends and significant others - are computed. MSPSS total scores range from 12 to 84, the higher score indicating greater satisfaction with overall support. The scale has been used among Israeli Arab and Jewish students and found reliable with Cronbach's alpha— 0.94' (Ben Ari and Gil, 2002).

For the entire sample, internal reliability as measured by Cronbach's *alpha* coefficient was consistently very satisfactory: GHQ-12, 0.85 (0.81 for Arabs and 0.85 for Jews); GSES, 0.92 (0.93 for Arabs and 0.91 for Jews); and for the different MSPSS subscales, 0.83-0.92 (0.86 for Arabs and 0.92 for Jews).

DATA ANALYSIS

All analyses were performed using the SPSS-14.0 software package. Chi-square statistics were employed to test the significance of differences in proportions. Two-tailed t-tests and Mann-Whitney two sample (non-matched) tests were used to define the significance of differences in means and standard deviations (SD) for normally and non-parametrically distributed scores, respectively. In addition, logistic regression analysis was performed to assess the contribution of Arab/Jewish-Israeli affiliation, controlling for selected variables, which differed significantly between the groups at the bivariate level. Significance in the logistic regression was assessed using the Wald statistical model. Hosmer and Lemeshow's goodness-of-fit (GOF) tests were used to examine the degree of fitness of the models (Hosmer et al., 2000).

Table 1. Arab- and Jewish-Israeli Patients by Demographic Characteristics

Characteristic	Arab-Israelis (n=75)	Jewish-Israelis (n=176)	Significance test
Gender (%)			
Male	45 (60.0)	101 (57.4)	χ^2=2.09, df=1, p=0.18
Female	30 (40.0)	75 (42.6)	
Age, mean±SD	35.8±11.1	37.3±13.3	$t_{1,222}$=0.64, p=0.52
Schooling, in years, (%)			
0-8	25 (39.1)	9 (5.3)	
9-12	37 (57.8)	115 (67.6)	χ^2=50.17, df=2, p<0.001
13+	2 (3.2)	46 (27.1)	
Mean±SD	9.5±2.2	12.4±2.6	t_{241}=8.08 p=0.001
Marital status (%)			
Single/divorced/widowed	26 (37.1)	100 (57.1)	
Married	44 (62.9)	75 (42.9)	χ^2=8.01, df=1, p<0.005
Employment (%)			
Full time	5 (6.7)	59 (33.7)	
Part time	10 (13.3)	34 (19.4)	χ^2=56.94, df=3, p<0.001
Unemployed	42 (56.0)	49 (28.0)	
Other (student, housewife, etc.)	18 (24.0)	33 (18.9)	
Religious observance			
Religious	71 (94.7)	60 (34.1)	χ^2=80.65, df=1, p<0.001
Secular	4 (5.3)	116 (65.9)	
Diagnosis (ICD-10)			
Organic & substance use disorders	7 (11.9)	3 (3.8)	
Schizophrenia	4 (6.8)	4 (5.1)	
Mood disorders	2 (3.4)	20 (25.2)	
Stress-related disorders	35 (59.3)	41 (51.9)	
Personality disorders	11 (18.6)	11 (14.0)	

To examine the emotional distress experienced by the two ethnic groups, multiple regression analyses were made, with GHQ-12 mean score as the dependent variable and ethnic affiliation (Arabs/Jews) as the variable under test. We controlled for potential confounders, including gender, years of education, marital status (married/unmarried), religious observance (religious/secular), ICD-10 diagnostic category (stress-related/other disorders), self-efficacy, and perceived total social support from family, friends, and significant others. Backward stepwise selection was performed on each model, removing variables with p>0.05 in order to find the most parsimonious model for the prediction of psychological distress.

RESULTS

Characteristics of the Arab- and Jewish-Israeli Groups

The two groups differed on several socio-demographic variables. More of the Arab-Israelis were married ($\chi^2=8.01$, df=1, p<0.005), they had less schooling ($\chi^2=59.17$, df=3, p<0.001), more were unemployed ($\chi^2=56.94$, df=3, p<0.001) and religious ($\chi^2=80.65$, df=1, p<0.001). The groups did not differ by gender ($\chi^2=0.38$; df=1, p=0.70) and by mean age (t=0.64, p=0.52).

A substantially higher proportion of the Arab-Israeli group was diagnosed with organic/substance use and personality disorders, while the frequency of mood disorders was higher among Jewish-Israeli subjects ($\chi^2=20.26$, df=4, p<0.01). No group differences were found in the diagnosis of schizophrenia and stress-related disorders.

Current Psychiatric Problems

The groups did not significantly differ on frequency of self-reported alcohol/drug use, behavioral problems and suicidal ideation as a reason for attending the clinics. However, compared with the Jewish-Israeli patients, the Arab-Israelis reported mood disturbances (64% vs. 38.1%; z=3.79) and emotional distress (68.4% vs. 89.7%, z=4.15, both p<0.001) significantly less often.

GHQ-12 emotional distress detection

Overall, Arabs scored significantly higher than Jews on the GHQ-12 (3.5±0.6 vs. 3.0±0.7; t=5.17, p<0.001). This was also the case when the GHQ-12 individual items were analyzed: on 9 of the 12 GHQ-12 items Arabs scored higher than Jews. Using a mean GHQ-12 score of 3 as cut-off point to distinguish cases of distress (3 and higher) from non-cases, we found 70.8% cases of distress in the Arab group versus 41.2% in the Jewish group (Man-Whitney two sample (non-matched) tests: z-value=4.32, p<0.0001).

Psychiatrist's Diagnosis

Table 2 presents the clinicians' ICD-10-based diagnoses and patient's self-reported problems (complaints) and their relation to GHQ-12 distress scores. The clinicians' intake diagnoses were available for 78.7% Arab and for 44.9% Jewish subjects. According to the psychiatrist' diagnosis, stress-related disorders was the most frequent ICD-10 diagnostic category in both groups (Arabs 46.7%, Jews 23.3%), while the least frequent categories were mood disorders among the Arab patients (1.7%), and organic/substance use disorders among the Jews (3.8%).

Compared to Jewish patients, Israeli-Arab patients had a higher rate of psychiatrist-detected ICD-10 stress-related disorders (46.7% vs. 23.3%), of organic/substance use disorders (9.3% vs. 1.7%) and of personality disorders (14.7% vs. 6.3%) but a lower rate of mood disorders (2.7% vs. 11.4%; χ^2=20.26, df=4, p<0.01). No significant difference in the detection rate for schizophrenia was found (2.3% vs. 5.3%).

Patients from both groups who were clinically diagnosed with organic/substance use disorders, schizophrenia and mood disorders did not differ on their mean GHQ-12 distress scores. Arabs with diagnoses of stress-related and, in particular, personality disorders, scored significantly higher distress scores than their Jewish counterparts (3.4±0.7 vs. 2.8±0.7, t=4.13 and 3.8±0.5 vs. 2.7±0.8, t=3.81, both p<0.001, respectively).

Table 2. Arab and Jewish Patients by Clinicians' Diagnoses, Patients' Self-Reported Mental Health Problems, and Distress Scores

	Arabs (N=75)			Jews N=176			z-value[†]	t-value[‡]
	N	%	GHQ Mean ± SD	N	%	GHQ Mean ± SD		
Clinical diagnoses (ICD-10)								
Organic & Substance use disorders	7	9.3	3.6±0.5	3	1.7	3.7±0.1	2.83**	0.46
Schizophrenia	4	5.3	3.7±0.8	4	2.3	3.2±1.4	1.26	0.69
Mood disorders	2	2.7	3.0±0.8	20	11.4	3.1±0.4	2.23*	0.46
Stress-related disorders	35	46.7	3.4±0.7	41	23.3	2.8±0.7	3.69***	4.13***
Personality disorders	11	14.7	3.8±0.5	11	6.3	2.7±0.8	2.16*	3.81***
Diagnosis pending	16	21.3	3.3±0.7	97	55.1	3.0±0.8	4.92***	1.19
Self-reported problems[#]	N=75			N=173				
Alcohol abuse	4	5.4	3.7±0.7	19	11.1	3.5±0.8	1.41	0.51
Mood disturbances	29	38.7	3.6±0.5	112	64.7	3.1±0.7	3.81***	3.60***
Suicide ideation	38	50.7	3.4±0.6	70	40.5	3.3±0.7	1.49	1.31
Behavior problems	32	42.7	3.7±0.6	56	32.4	3.3±0.6	1.56	2.46*
Emotional distress	27	36.0	3.4±0.5	94	54.3	3.1±0.7	2.65**	1.96*
Phobias	25	33.3	3.5±0.7	63	36.6	3.2±0.7	0.47	2.00*

[#] More than one problem could be reported.
[†] Mann–Whitney two sample (non-matched) test. [‡] Two-tailed t-test.
* p<0.05, ** p<0.01, *** p<0.001

Self-Reported Problems (Complaints)

According to the self-report checklist of complaints, the most frequent problems for these applicants for outpatient care were mood disturbances for the Jews and suicide ideation for the Arabs (64.7% and 50%, respectively) while the least reported problem was alcohol abuse for both groups (11.1% and 5.4%, respectively). The groups did not significantly differ in their self-reported rates of alcohol/drug use, behavioral problems, and suicidal ideation. There were significant differences with regard to mood disturbances and experienced emotional distress, which were higher among Jews than among Arabs (64.7% versus 38.7%; z=3.79, p<0.001, and 54.3% versus 36%, z=4.15, p<0.001, respectively).

Although the Jews reported mood disturbances and emotional distress more friquently than the Arabs did, Arabs reporting these conditions scored higher on the GHQ-12 than their Jewish counterparts (3.6±0.5 versus 3.1±0.7, t=3.60, p<0.001 and 3.4±0.5 versus 3.1±0.7, t=1.96, p<0.05).

Table 3. Arab and Jewish Outpatients by Self-Efficacy and Perceived Social Support from Family, Friends, and Significant Others

Measure	N	Arabs	N	Jews	t-value	(df) [a]
GSES [b]	68	2.0±0.6	153	2.4±0.7	3.89***	(1,219)
MSPSS, [c] total score	64	46.4±20.3	149	57.4±18.4	3.74***	(1,211)
Family support	72	18.0±7.8	165	19.8±7.5	1.62	(1,235)
Friends support	68	12.2±7.9	159	17.6±7.7	4.76***	(1,225)
Significant Others support	68	16.7±7.7	155	20.0±6.9	3.04**	(1,221)

[a] Two-tailed t-tests: * - p<.05; ** - p<.01; *** - p<.001
[b] General Self-Efficacy Scale
[c] Multidimensional Scale of Perceived Social Support

**Table 4. Parsimonious Model for Predicting GHQ Distress Scores
from Demographic, Clinical and Psychosocial Variables**

Independent Variables	Standardized Estimation (β)	t-Value (β=0)	Probability Level	Total % Variance Accounted For
Predictor Variables				
Self-Efficacy	-.458	8.47	.001	27.1
Ethnic Group (Arab/Jewish)	.233	3.56	.001	8.8
Social Support (Total Score)	-.136	2.50	.013	7.2
Religious Observance (Religious/Secular)	-.128	2.03	.044	0.7
Variables Removed				
Education (Years)	.002	.039	.969	-
Diagnosis (Stress-Related/Other)	.042	.790	.430	-
Marital Status (Married/Unmarried)	.050	.923	.357	-
Gender	-.087	-1.628	.105	-

R^2=0.33; Adjusted R^2=0.32; $F_{4,251}$=30.83, p<0.0001

Other Psychosocial Measures

Table 3 shows that Jewish subjects scored higher than Arabs with regard to feelings of self-efficacy (t=3.89, p<0.001), the total level of perceived social support (t=3.74, p<0.001), support from friends (t=4.76, p<0.001) and from significant others (t=3.04, p<0.01). No between-group differences were found in perceived family support (t=1.62, p>0.10).

Predictors of Psychological Distress

Table 4 presents a summary of the multiple regression analysis used here to examine the relationship between emotional distress, as summarized by the GHQ-12 mean score, (the dependent variable) and ethnic affiliation (Arabs/Jews), while controlling for other independent variables. In a reduced version of the initial model, which included 8 independent variables (ethnic group, gender, years of education, marital status, religious observance, ICD-10 diagnostic category, self-efficacy, and social support aggregated from family, friends, and significant others), only 4 variables were associated with a higher likelihood of psychological distress. Of these four, three— low sense of self-efficacy, ethnicity (being Arab), and insufficient social support accounted for 27.1%, 8.8%, and 7.2% of the total variance in the GHQ-12 distress scores (R^2=0.33; Adjusted R^2=0.32; $F_{4,251}$=30.83, p<0.0001). Although significant, the contribution of religious observance (religious/secular) to this model was negligible (0.7% of the variance).

Table 5. Reasons for Treatment Delay, Pathway to Clinic Care, Source of Referral to Psychiatric Clinic, and Current Psychiatric Problems

	Arab-Israelis N=75	Jewish-Israelis N=176	z-value#
Reason for treatment lag^			
Lack of resources	24 (31.6)	17 (9.7)	4.30***
Other-than-psychiatric attribution	41 (53.9)	59 (33.7)	3.06**
Stigma	45 (59.2)	60 (34.3)	3.68***
First agent contacted			
Social network	6 (7.9)	62 (35.4)	4.51***
Family doctor, non-psychiatrist	35 (46.0)	37 (21.1)	4.01***
Mental health services	9 (11.8)	21 (12.0)	0.03
Social worker/INII agent/ clerk/army physician	8 (10.5)	25 (14.3)	0.81
Source of referral			
Self-referral	7 (9.2)	50 (28.6)	3.36***
Family member/friend/neighbor/ employer/religious authority	9 (11.8)	33 (18.8)	1.37
Family doctor/non-psychiatrist	55 (72.4)	89 (50.8)	3.17**
Social worker/NIII agent/ police/court	6 (7.8)	5 (2.8)	1.79
Current psychiatric problems			
Mood disturbances	29 (38.1)	112 (64.0)	3.79***
Suicide ideation	38 (50.0)	70 (40.0)	1.47
Behavior problems	32 (42.1)	56 (32.0)	1.54
Emotional distress/unreasonable fears	52 (68.4)	157 (89.7)	4.15***
Alcohol/substance abuse	4 (5.3)	19 (10.8)	1.41

^ Subjects were allowed to give more than one reason
# Mann-Whitney two-sample (non-matched) test, two-tailed
* $p<0.05$; ** $p< 0.01$; *** $p< 0.001$
INII = the National Insurance Institute of Israel

Treatment Lag

The length of treatment lag in the total sample varied from 1.5 months to 37 years (mean=4.7 years, SD=6.7). The median number of years elapsed between onset of disorder and initial treatment visit to a mental health specialist was three years for the Arab-Israeli group, and half that (1.5 years) for the Jewish-Israelis (Yates' corrected χ^2=4.00, df=1, p <0.05). No other study variable was associated with treatment lag.

Table 6. Arab-Israeli and Jewish-Israeli Patients by Attitudes to Aspects of the Treatment of Mental Disorders

Attitude	Arab-Israelis	Jewish-Israelis	Significance test
Treatability of mental disorders	N=72	N=141	
All treatable	19 (26.4)	17 (12.1)	
Most treatable	31 (43.1)	100 (70.9)	χ^2= 16.22, df=2, p<0.001
None treatable	22 (30.6)	24 (17.0)	
Treatability of one's own mental problem	N=74	N=166	
Quite treatable	24 (32.4)	103 (62.0)	
Partly treatable	13 (17.6)	31 (18.7)	χ^2= 25.49, df=3, p<0.0001
Not treatable	10 (13.5)	10 (6.0)	
Not sure	27 (36.5)	22 (13.3)	
Type of treatment needed	N=74	N=169	
Only medication	7 (9.5)	16 (9.5)	
Only psychotherapy	13 (17.6)	47 (27.8)	
Medication and psychotherapy	16 (21.6)	63 (37.3)	χ^2=25.65, df=4, p<0.0001
Does not know	38 (51.4)	43 (25.4)	
Fear of medication	N=73	N=167	
Much	27 (37.0)	55 (33.0)	
Some	12 (16.4)	55 (32.9)	χ^2=12.82, df=3, p<.01
Not at all	18 (24.7)	43 (25.7)	
Not sure	16 (21.9)	14 (8.4)	
Reason for fear of medication*			
Habituation	43 (70.5)	71 (48.3)	χ^2=6.45, df=1, p<0.01
Mind control	11 (18.0)	35 (23.8)	χ^2=0.83, df=1, ns.
Adverse effects	14 (23.0)	53 (36.1)	χ^2=3.93, df=1, ns.
Other	7 (11.5)	20 (13.6)	χ^2=0.17, df=1, ns
Time required for treatment	N=74	N=150	
One week	2 (2.7)	3 (2.0)	
One month	3 (4.1)	9 (6.0)	χ^2=11.38, df=3, p<0.05
Six months and over	2 (2.7)	24 (16.0)	
Does not know	67 (90.5)	114 (76.0)	
Familiarity with someone in psychiatric care	N=73	N=167	
Yes	26 (35.6)	87 (52.1)	
No	38 (52.1)	66 (39.5)	χ^2=10.12, df=2, p<0.01
Not sure	9 (12.3)	14 (8.4)	

* Subjects allowed giving more than one reason.

Reasons Given for Treatment Lag

The groups differed significantly with regard to the reasons given for the delay in treatment. Arab-Israelis reported more often than Jewish-Israelis, lack of instrumental resources (e.g., time, money) (31.6% vs. 9.7%; z-value=4.30, p<0.001) and gave an other-than-psychiatric attribution for the presenting problem (e.g., "my problem is non-psychiatric" or "the problem will resolve itself") (53.9% vs. 33.7%; z=3.06; p<0.01), as well as negative attitudes towards the treatment of mental disorders (e.g., negative advice from family, friends or a religious leader about seeking professional help, lack of confidence in psychiatry and the effectiveness of psychiatric medication) (59.2% vs.34.3%; z=3.68, p<0.001).

Help-Seeking and Referral Sources

Arab-Israeli patients preferred to turn to family doctors or other non-psychiatric medical professionals (46%), while Jewish-Israeli patients more often sought help from members of their social network before consulting a psychiatrist (35.4%). Accordingly, among Arab-Israelis it was the family doctor/non-psychiatrist physician who more often referred the subjects to the psychiatric clinic than was the case for the Jewish-Israeli group (72.4% vs. 50.8%, z-value=3.17, p<0.01), while the Jewish-Israelis had a higher frequency of self-referral (28.6% vs. 9.2%; z=3.36, p<0.001).

Attitudes to Treatment of Mental Disorders

The Jewish-Israeli group was significantly more optimistic with regard to the treatment of most mental disorders than its counterpart (70.9% vs. 43.1%; χ^2=16.22, p<0.001). They were also more positive as to the susceptibility to treatment of their own mental problem (62% vs. 32.4%; χ^2=25.49, p<0.001).

Type of treatment needed

We found significant group differences in views on the type of treatment needed. While Arab-Israeli patients more frequently expressed no preference (51.4% vs. 25.4%), the Jewish-Israeli patients preferred psychotherapy (27.8% vs. 17.6%) or a combination of psychotherapy and medication (37.3% vs. 21.6%; χ^2=25.65, df=3, p<0.001).

Fear of psychiatric medication

In general, the Jewish-Israeli patients reported significantly more fear of taking medication than the Arab-Israeli patients (χ^2=12.82, df=3, p<0.001). Among the specific reasons for such fear, Arab-Israelis more frequently than Jewish-Israelis cited the risk of habituation to the medication (49.2% vs. 30.6%; χ^2=6.45, df=1, p<0.01), while the Jews tended to be more afraid of adverse reactions to medication.

Time required for treatment

The majority of patients had no clue as to the time required to treat the presenting problem. The Arab-Israeli group thought more time was needed than the Jewish-Israelis (Arab, 90.5% vs. Jews, 76%; χ^2=11.38, df=3, p<0.05).

Knowing someone in psychiatric care

While 52.1% of the Jewish-Israeli patients reported knowing someone who had received psychiatric treatment, the same proportion of Arab-Israeli patients reported not knowing anybody like that (χ^2=12.82, df=3, p<0.01).

Table 7. Logistic Regression Model of Factors Associated with Ethnicity

Predictor variables	Goodness-of-fit	Wald χ^2	df	p
Schooling years	43.97	25.61	1	0.001
Treatability of one's own mental problem	30.59	20.51	3	0.001
Treatability of mental disorders in general	15.89	12.31	2	0.002
Other-than-psychiatric attribution of mental symptoms	6.41	5.80	1	0.016

Adjusted R^2=0.42; Likelihood ratioχ^2=84.929; d.f.=7; p<0.001
Prediction success rate=0.84

Multivariate Analyses

A multivariate logistic regression analysis was conducted to control for confounding effects when studying group differences (Table 7). Only 4 of the 17 independent variables were found to be significantly associated with one ethnic group or the other. These were: schooling (goodness-of-fit (GOF)= 43.97, Wald χ^2 = 25.61, df=1, p=0.001); treatment of mental disorders, both in general (GOF=15.89; Wald χ^2 = 12.31, df=2;p=0.002) and for oneself

(GOF=30.59; Wald χ^2 = 20.51, df=3, p=0.001); and other-than-psychiatric attribution of mental symptoms (GOF=6.41; Wald χ^2 =5.80, df=1, p=0.016). This model (Adjusted R^2=0.42; Likelihood ratio χ^2=84.93; df=7; p<0.001) was able to correctly classify 84% of the patients as belonging either to the Arab-Israeli or the Jewish-Israeli group.

DISCUSSION

This study reported here showed that, compared to their Israeli-Jewish counterparts, Israeli-Arabs, seeking help for the first time in their lives for mental health problems from psychiatric outpatient clinics, had significantly higher emotional distress as measured by the GHQ-12 scores and a higher rate of psychiatrist-detected ICD-10 stress-related disorders. However, they reported a lower rate of emotional distress and symptoms of mood disturbances as a reason for seeking healthcare. Moreover, they apparently have significantly less psychosocial resources to cope with stress, such as feelings of self-efficacy and social support from friends and significant others. The multiple regression analysis confirmed the association of emotional distress with ethnic affiliation (being Arab) and low feelings of self-efficacy and total social support.

For both groups, Jews and Arabs, the rate of detection by the GHQ-12 was higher than for the other two detection methods used. However, there were significant cultural differences in the detection of distress by the patients themselves and by their psychiatrists. The GHQ-12 detection rate was in agreement with the psychiatrists' diagnoses but not with patients' identification of emotional distress and disturbance. These results suggest a significant difference between the ethnic groups according to which of the three methods of case detection is used. Israeli Arabs seem to be prone to complain less than Jews of emotional distress, which, however, both psychiatrist and GHQ-12 detect. This clear discrepancy may be explained by culturally shared health beliefs, whereby in Arab culture emotional symptoms (fears, worries, low spirits) are attributed to weakness of personality or weakness of religious faith. Depressed people can readily accept and internalize this notion and so not self-report emotional problems.

How to Interpret These Findings?

One possible explanation is that Israeli Arabs, who are usually more distant from services, may need to be feeling higher distress than Jews before they will seek psychiatric care. Another explanation is that minority status and associated lower socioeconomic status may be responsible for the higher levels of distress found among Arab applicants, independent of their help-seeking attitudes and behavior. Another factor making application more likely to the formal service system, in particular long-term care services, is the change in the availability and capacity of the Arab informal support system to address these increasing needs (Azaiza and Brodsky, 2003).

Specific health belief systems may also influence the way patients interact with a psychiatrist. Culture makes the Arab patient–doctor relationship triangular rather than dyadic/linear, as there is two-way communication between patient, doctor and family. Although some degree of personal independence is allowed, interpersonal concern, interdependence and minimal 'social distances' are the norm in Arabian families. For example, the doctor is not expected to encourage adolescents to achieve Western-type full independence from their parents. Not only is this culturally undesirable but there are also no socio-economic provisions for adolescents to live away from their families. Arab doctors encourage this interdependent group ego. The Arab family runs the affairs of its healthy and unhealthy members alike. The decision to seek the help of professionals or traditional healers is one made by the family (El-Islam, 2005).

The psychosocial resources scores (self-efficacy and social support) confirm that the finding of higher emotional distress among Arabs compared to Jews is not an artifact. Stress theory suggests that social and emotional support may serve as a major resource for coping with stressful situations (Lazarus and Folkman, 1984). Members of minority groups may suffer not only from the distress inherent in their status but also from alienation and lack of social support (Comino et al., 2001). Although the Arab population in Israel is currently undergoing a modernization process, it is still dominated by traditional values and ideology. Israeli Arabs generally maintain their separateness by exhibiting low motivation towards integration into Israeli society, even in academic settings (Sagiv and Shwartz, 1998). Traditional networks of social support do not provide a sufficient buffer against distress (Ben-Ari, 2002). These findings are in line with other recent studies on how minority groups deal with the negative effects of stress (Gillock and Reyes, 1999). Arab students, for example, turn to partners and best friends as the primary sources of social support in emotionally stressful situations, rather than to members of the family of origin. In this way partners and friends help bridge the gap between tradition and modernization. Reflecting this situation, our findings show that the Arab attendees who seek help from formal psychiatric services report insufficient social support from friends and significant others, while reporting a level of social support from family no different from that of the Jewish patients.

Reverse causality, namely the likelihood that a low perception of social support results from current psychopathology cannot be ruled out. However, this seems unlikely because a diagnosis of stress-related disorder was removed from the regression model as non-statistically significant, whereas low social support was found to be a markedly significant predictor of distress

Compared to their Jewish-Israeli counterparts, Arab-Israeli patients showed a two-fold delay in their initial treatment contact. Many variables distinguished between the groups, and each of them, alone or in combination with others, could contribute to treatment delay. Logistic regression analysis showed that the relationship between treatment delay and a lower level of schooling, other-than-psychiatric attribution of mental symptoms, and more pessimistic attitudes to the treatment of mental disorders both in general and for oneself was mediated by ethnic affiliation (being Arab). Most of these factors can be addressed through mental health education programs (Merinder, 2000).

Our findings suggest that the central link in this constellation of factors is lack of schooling, which leads to ignorance about mental disorders and treatment possibilities. The lack of such information easily gives rise to negative (stigmatizing) attitudes to people with mental disorders and to the likelihood of successful treatment. The longer delay for the Arab-Israeli group was related to their negative attitudes. Correspondingly, the shorter delay for the Jewish-Israeli group might be imputed to their more optimistic view on the treatability of mental disorders, and their expectation—correct or incorrect—as to the length of treatment.

Mulvany et al (2001) have shown that whereas social class of origin does not seem to be an important risk factor for schizophrenia it does partially determine patients getting treatment at a later age. Thus, the relation between low social class at birth and poor outcome may be at least partially mediated through treatment delay. In our study, low socioeconomic status (SES), to the extent that it is captured by socio-demographic characteristics, may have led those married and unemployed and with lower schooling level to delay seeking the social support of mental health treatment. This reason for delayed presentation for treatment, in combination with indications of lower SES, was found more frequently in the Arab than the Jewish sub-sample.

The stigmatization of psychiatric problems and the psychological barriers to seeking help for mental dysfunction or substance abuse are thought to be important determinants of the undertreatment of psychiatric disorders (Sirey, 2001; Lauber et al., 2006; Seedat et al., 2002; Alonso et al., 2004; Ak-Krenawi et al., 2004). Negative preconceptions may also result in non-compliance with beneficial psychiatric treatments, perceived as a sign of weakness and inability to cope with misfortune. This is particularly true in Arab culture, where emotional symptoms (fears, worries, low spirits) are attributed to weakness of personality or weakness of religious faith (El-Islam, 2005). In the present study, the Arab-Israeli patients cited stigma substantially more frequently than their Jewish counterparts as a reason for treatment delay. This finding could be explained by significant differences found between the study subsamples with regard to religious affiliation. As previous studies have showed negative (stigmatizing) attitudes to mental disorders and treatment are expressed and mental health service utilization is lowered among religious communities (Cinnirella and Loewenthal, 1999; Feinberg, 2005). These reasons fit also to explain lower psychotropic drug use among Arabs (Al Krenawi et al., 2004; El-Islam, 2005) and, probably, other religious minorities in Israel (Daie et al., 1992; Iancu et al., 1998).

In other contexts, even health professionals have portrayed psychiatric treatment as cosmetic and indicative of a superficial life style. Other psychiatric practices, such as electroconvulsive therapy, involuntary hospitalization, the treatment of children with stimulants and suicide prevention, are also subject to stigma and, for some groups, constitute breaches of individual autonomy and freedom. In line with such attitudes to psychiatric treatment and practices, we found that the Arab-Israeli patients sought help for their mental problems more frequently than their Jewish counterparts from family doctors and non-psychiatric medical professionals. It is possible that presenting their problems first to general practitioners could prolong the time that elapses until their first psychiatric contact due to inadequate and time-consuming attempts to have their psychiatric problems treated by a non-specialist (Gater et al., 2005; Nutt et al., 2006).

The findings of previous studies that severity of disorder is associated with probability of treatment and shorter delay (Wang et al., 2002; Wang et al., 2004; Wells et al., 1995; Leaf et al., 1988; Demyttenaere et al., 2004) were supported by the present study. In particular, we found that compared with their Jewish counterparts, fewer Arab attendees were diagnosed by a psychiatrist with a mood disorder and fewer Arab-Israelis self-reported mood disturbances or experienced emotional distress.

Although the Jewish attendees reported more often than Arab patients some fear of taking psychiatric medication, the groups gave different reasons for this fear: Jews were afraid of medication side-effects, while Arabs feared addiction. It is possible that having the same attitude to psychiatric medication as to illicit drugs may postpone treatment-seeking among the Arab group.

Previous studies on attitudes to mental disorders have shown that respondents who have had personal contact with a mentally ill person are more willing to interact with a person in psychiatric care (Chung et al., 2001; Ponizovsky et al., 2003) and that the more the respondents are familiar with psychiatric treatment, the less stigmatization they display (Angermeyer and Matschinger, 2005). Consistently with these studies, we found that Jews as a group, who more often acknowledged knowing someone who had received psychiatric treatment, also delayed seeking treatment less. It is plausible that their more frequent familiarity with someone in psychiatric treatment enabled them to form a more optimistic view of the successful treatment of mental disorders in general and their own mental problem in particular. In line with this positive thinking, the Jews gave more differential preferences with regard to the type of treatment needed in their particular case. Though both groups were uncertain about the treatment time their mental problem required, the Jews reported such uncertainty less frequently.

There are several limitations that need to be kept in mind in interpreting the results of these studies. The first is that attendees were asked to retrospectively recall and date the first onset of their disorder. Recall bias could overestimate treatment lag. However, this recall failure would be common for all participants and, hence, cannot explain the substantial between-group difference in treatment delay. We are uncertain whether our questions affected recall accuracy of the date of the first appearance of symptoms, but significantly smaller treatment delay was found in this study than in previous surveys using other instruments (Wang et al., 2004; Merinder, 2000; Knauper et al., 1999). Second, a relatively small sample-size limited the number of variables we could examine in order to avoid multiple comparisons generating spurious findings. Third, both small number of non-Muslims in the Arab subgroup and immigrants in the Jewish subgroup precluded comparisons of inter-religious and inter-cultural factors, which could potentially influence help-seeking patterns and treatment delay.

In addition, as a matter of convenience the Israeli-Jewish group included several Russian-born Jewish immigrants, who might differ from Israel-born

Jews with regards to psychopathology and psychosocial resources. The methodology did not allow psychiatrists not to know their patient's responses to the GHQ-12, although it was believed that they have made their diagnosis independently. The psychiatrist reading the patient section of the questionnaire would have had the effect increasing, not decreasing, the agreement between patient self-report and psychiatrist detection. Third, there was no 'gold standard' such as the Composite International Diagnostic Interview (Wittchen et al., 1991) to confirm the diagnoses. Likewise, the GHQ-12 and self-report items were based on western conceptualizations of emotional distress. Finally, although we did not test diagnostic agreement between the Israeli Jewish and Arab clinicians who participated in the study, we suggest that there is satisfactory concordance between diagnoses made by them, as they are all products of the Israeli medical training system (Greenberg and Cohen, 1999).

CLINICAL IMPLICATIONS

The presented data may help in identifying difficulties to detection of common symptoms of anxiety and depression comprising emotional distress among members of the ethnic minority first attending mental health clinics in Israel. The clinical implication of the findings of this study are that it may be possible to improve psychiatrist detection of emotional distress and mood disturbances among Arab patients by the physician relying on GHQ-12 scores rather than on the patient's complaints or subjective sense of health.

CONCLUSION

The results of this study suggest that the ethnic background of patients brings about substantial variation in the rates of detection of emotional distress and symptoms. This variation can be predicted by lower senses of self-efficacy and social support among Israeli Arabs, as compared to Israeli Jews.

In conclusion, the longer treatment lag this study found was mostly associated with potentially modifiable knowledge and attitudes to mental disorders and treatment. What is needed, therefore, is educational programs tailored to the different consumer sectors and the different community gatekeepers of access to psychiatric care, programs designed to raise confidence in the treatability of mental disorders and so shorten treatment lag.

Further research into treatment delay and the factors associated with it, in a wider national framework, is also clearly warranted.

REFERENCES

Abdel-Khalek AM. Internal consistency of an Arabic adaptation of the Beck Depression Inventory in four Arab countries. *Psychol Rep* 1998;82:264–266.

Abou-Saleh MT, Ghubash R, Daradkeh TK. A1 Ain Community Psychiatric Survey. I. Prevalence and socio-demographic correlates. *Soc Psychiatry Psychiatr Epidemiol* 2001;36:20–28.

Abyad A. Health care for older persons: A country profile — Lebanon. *J Am Geriatr Soc* 2001;49:1366–1370.

Al-Krenawi A, Graham JR, Dean YZ, Eltaiba N. Crossnational study of attitudes towards seeking professional elp: Jordan, United Arab Emirates (UAE) and Arabs in Israel. *Int J Soc Psychiatry* 2004;50:102–114.

Alonso J, Angermeyer MC, Bernert S, Bruffaerts R, Brugha TS, Bryson H, de Girolamo G, Graaf R, Demyttenaere K, Gasquet I, Haro JM, Katz SJ, Kessler RC, Kovess V, Lepine JP, Ormel J, Polidori G, Russo LJ Vilagut G, Almansa J, Arbabzadeh-Bouchez S, Autonell J, BernalM, Buist-Bouwman MA, Codony M, Domingo-Salvany A, Ferrer M, Joo SS, Martinez-Alonso M, Matschinger H, Mazzi F, Morgan Z, Morosini P, Palacin C, Romera B, Taub N, Vollebergh WA; ESEMeD/MHEDEA 2000 Investigators, European Study of the Epidemiology of Mental Disorders SEMeD) Project. Use of mental health services in Europe: Results from the European Study of the Epidemiology of Mental Disorders (ESEMeD) project. *Acta Psychiatr Scand* 2004;109(suppl 420):47–54.

Amaddeo F, Zambello F, Tansella M, Thournicroft G. Accessibility and pathways to psychiatric care in a community-based mental health system. *Soc Psychiatry Psychiatr Epidemiol* 2001;36:500–507.

Andrews G, Issakidis C, Carter G. Shortfall in mental health service utilisation. *Br J Psychiatry* 2001;179: 417–425.

Angermeyer MC, Matschinger H, Riedel-Heller SG. Whom to ask for help in case of a mental disorder? Preferences of the lay public. *Soc Psychiatry Psychiatr Epid* 1999;34:202–210.

Angermeyer MC, Matschinger H. The stigma of mental illness in Germany: A trend analysis. *Int J Soc Psychiatry* 2005;51:276–284.

Azaiza F, Brodsky J. The aging of Israel's Arab population: Needs, existing responses, and dilemmas in the development of services for a society in transition. *Isr Med Assoc J* 2003;5:383–386.

Barnes TR, Hutton SB, Chapman MJ, Mustatsa S, Puri BK, Joyce EM. West London first-episode study of schizophrenia: Clinical correlates of duration of untreated psychosis. *Br J Psychiatry* 2000;177:207–211.

Becker S, Al Zaid K, Al Faris E. Screening for somatization and depression in Saudi Arabia: A validation study of the PHQ in primary care. *Int J Psychiatry Med* 2002;32:271–283.

Ben-Ari A, Gil S. Traditional support systems: Are they sufficient in a culturally diverse academic environment? *Br J Soc Work* 2002;32:629–638.

Ben-Ari A. Support functions and utilization of sources of social support: Views from Israeli Jewish and Arab students. *Fam Soc* 2002;83:93–101.

Bijl RV, de Graaf R, Hiripi E, Kessler RC, Kohn R, Offord DR, Ustun TB, Vicente B, Vollebergh WA, Walters EE, Wittchen HU. The prevalence of treated and untreated mental disorders in five countries. *Health Aff* (Millwood) 2003;22:122–133.

Carbone S, Harrigan S, McGorry PD. Duration of untreated psychosis and 12 month outcome in first episode psychosis: The impact of treatment approach. *Acta Psychiatr Scand* 1999;100:96–104.

Cheung SK, Sun SY. Assessment of optimistic self-beliefs:Further validation of the Chinese version of theGeneral Self-Efficacy Scale. *Psychol Rep* 1999;85:1221–1224.

Chung KF, Chen EY, Liu CS. University students' attitudes to mental patients and psychiatric treatment. *Int J Soc Psychiatry* 2001;47:63–72. 40. Ponizovsky A, Grinshpoon A, Sasson R, Baidani- Auerbach A, Ben Eliezer D, Shershevsky Y. Knowledge and attitudes about mental disorders among principals of adult education schools. *Isr J Psychiatry Relat Sci* 2003;40:283–289.

Cinnirella M, Loewenthal KM. Religious and ethnic group influences on beliefs about mental illness: A qualitative interview study. *Br J Med Psychol* 1999;72: 505–524.

Comino EJ, Silove D, Manicavasagar V, Harris E, HarrisMF. Agreement in symptoms of anxiety and depression between patients and GPs: The influence of ethnicity. *Fam Pract* 2001;18:71–77.

Daie N, Wiztum E, Mark M, Rabinowitz S. The belief in the transmigration of souls: Psychotherapy of a Druze patient with severe anxiety reaction. *Br J Med Psychol* 1992;65:119–130.

Demyttenaere K, Bruffaerts R, Posada-Villa J, Gasquet I, Kovess V, Lepine JP, Angermeyer MC, Bernert S, de Girolamo G, Morosini P, Polidori G, Kikkawa T, Kawakami N, Ono Y, Takeshima T, Uda H, Karam EG, Fayyad JA, Karam AN, Mneimneh ZN, Medina-Mora ME, Borges G, Lara C, de Graaf R, Ormel J, Gureje O, Shen Y, Huang Y, ZhangM, Alonso J, Haro JM, Vilagut G, Bromet EJ, Gluzman S, Webb C, Kessler RC, Merikangas KR, Anthony JC, Von KorffMR,Wang PS, Brugha TS,

Aguilar-Gaxiola S, Lee S, Heeringa S, Pennell BE, Zaslavsky AM, Ustun TB, Chatterji S; WHO World Mental Health Survey Consortium. Prevalence, severity, and unmet need for treatment of mental disorders in the World Health Organization World Mental Health Surveys. *J Am Med Assoc* 2004;291:2581–2590.

Denton M, Prus S, Walters V. Gender differences in health: A Canadian study of the psychosocial, structural and behavioral determinants of health. *Soc Sci Med* 2004;58:2585–2600.

Dohrenwend BP, Shrout PE, Egri G, Mendelsohn FS. Nonspecific psychological distress and other dimensions of psychopathology. Measures for use in the general population. *Arch Gen Psychiatry* 1980;37:1229–1236.

Drake RJ, Haley CJ, Akhtar S, Lewis SW. Causes and consequences of duration of untreated psychosis in schizophrenia. *Br J Psychiatry* 2000;177:511–515.

El-Islam MF. Some cultural aspects of the Arab patient-doctor relationship *Int Psychiatry* 2005;7:18–20.

Feinberg SS. Issues in the psychopharmacologic assessment and treatment of the orthodox Jewish patient. *CNS Spectrum* 2005;10:954–965.

Fry PS, Debats DL. Self-efficacy beliefs as predictors of loneliness and psychological distress in older adults. *Int J Aging Hum Dev* 2002;55:233–269.

Gater R, JordanovaV, Maric N, Alikaj V, Bajs M, Cavic T, Dimitrov H, Iosub D, Mihai A, Szalontay AS, Helmchen H, Sartorius N. Pathways to psychiatric care in Eastern Europe. *Br J Psychiatry* 2005;186:529–535.

Ghubash R, Daradkeh TK, Ghubash R, Daradkeh TK, Al-Muzafari SM, Al-Manssori ME, Abou-Saleh MT. Al-Ain community psychiatric survey IV: Socio-cultural changes (traditionality-liberalism) and prevalence of psychiatric disorders. *Soc Psychiatry Psychiatr Epidemiol* 2001;36:565–570.

Ghubash R, Hamdi E, Bebbington P. The Dubai Community Psychiatric Survey: I. Prevalence and socio-demographic correlates. *Soc Psychiatry Psychiatr Epidemiol* 1992;27:53–61.

Gillock KL, Reyes O. Stress, support, and academic performance of urban, low-income, Mexican-American adolescent. *J Youth Adol* 1999;28:259–282.

Goldberg DP, Williams P. *A users' guide to the general health questionnaire: GHQ.* Windsor: NFER-NELSON, 1988.

Greenberg D, Cohen R. A survey of the teaching of undergraduate psychiatry in Israel. *Isr J Psychiatry Relat Sci* 1999;36:282–290.

Grzywacz JG, Almeida DM, Neupert SD, Ettner SL. Socioeconomic status and health: A micro-level analysis of exposure and vulnerability to daily stressors. *J Health Soc Behav* 2004;45:1–16.

Ho BC, Alicata D, Ward J, Moser DJ, O'Leary DS, Arndt S, Andreasen NC. Untreated initial psychosis: Relation to cognitive deficits and brain morphology in first-episode schizophrenia. *Am J Psychiatry* 2003;160: 142–148.

Ho BC, Andreasen NC. Long delays in seeking treatmentfor schizophrenia. *Lancet* 2001;357:898–840.

Hosmer Jr DW, Lemeshow S. *Applied logistic regression*. New York: Wiley, 2000.

Iancu I, Spivak B, Mester R, Weizman A. Belief in transmigration of the soul and psychopathology in Israeli Druze. A culture-sensitive psychotherapeutic approach. *Psychopathology* 1998;31:52–58.

Idel M, Melamed S, Merlob P, Yahav J, Hendel T, Kaplan B. Influence of a merger on nurses' emotional well-being: The importance of self-efficacy and emotional reactivity. *J Nurs Manag* 2003;11:59–63.

Kessler RC, Olfson M, Berglund PA. Patterns and predictors of treatment contact after first onset of psychiatric disorders. *Am J Psychiatry* 1998;155:62–69.

Kessler RC, Price RH, Wortman CB. Social factors in psychopathology: Stress, social support, and coping processes. *Ann Rev Psychol* 1985;36:531–572.

Knauper B, Cannell CF, Schwarz N, Bruce ML, Kessler RC. Improving accuracy of major depression age of onset reports in the U.S. National Comorbidity Survey. *IntJ Meth Psychiatr Res* 1999;8:39–48.

Kohn R, Saxena S, Levav I, Saraceno B. Treatment gap in mental health care. *Bull World Health Org* 2004;82: 858–866.

Kornblith AB, Herndon JE 2nd, Zuckerman E, Viscoli CM, Horwitz RI, Cooper MR, Harris L, Tkaczuk KH, Perry MC, Budman D, Norton LC, Holland J. Cancer and Leukemia Group B. Social support as a buffer to the psychological impact of stressful life events in women with breast cancer. *Cancer* 2001;91:443–454.

Larsen TK, Johannessen JO, Opjordsmoen S. First-episode schizophrenia with long duration of untreated psychosis. Pathways to care. *Br J Psychiatry* 1998;172(Suppl):45–52.

Larsen TK, McGlashan TH, Moe LC. First-episode schizophrenia: I. Early course parameters. *Schizophr Bull* 1996;22:241–256.

Larsen TK, Moe LC, Vibe-Hansen L, Johannessen JO. Premorbid functioning versus duration of untreated psychosis in 1 year outcome in first-episode psychosis. *Schizophr Res* 2000;45:1–9.

Lauber C, Nordt C, Haker H, Falcato L, Rossler W. Community psychiatry: Results of a public opinion survey. *Int J Soc Psychiatry* 2006;52:234–242.

Laukkala T, Isometsa E, Hamalainen J, Heikkinen M, Lindeman S, Aro H. Antidepressant treatment of depression in the Finnish general population. *Am J Psychiatry* 2001;158:2077–2079.

Lazarus R S, Folkman S. *Stress, appraisal, and coping.* New York: Springer, 1984.

Leaf PJ, Bruce ML, Tischler GL, Freeman DH Jr, Weissman MM, Myers JK. Factors affecting the utilization of specialty and general medical mental health services. *Med Care* 1988;26:9–26.

Levav I. *Psychiatric and Behavioral Disorders in Israel: From Epidemiology to Mental Health Action.* Gefen Publishing House, Jerusalem, 2009.

Levav I, Al-Krenawi A, Ifrah A, Geraisy N, Grinshpoon A, Khwaled R, Levinson D. Common mental disorders among Arab-Israelis: findings from the Israel NationalHealth Survey. *Isr J Psychiatry Relat Sci* 2007;44:104-113.

Levav I, Grinshpoon A. Mental health services in Israel. *Int Psychiatry* 2004;4:10–14.

Loebel AD, Lieberman JA, Alvir JMJ, Mayerhoff DI,Geisler SH, Szymanski SR. Duration of psychosis and outcome in first-episode schizophrenia. *Am J Psychiatry* 1992;149:1183–1188.

May S. Patient satisfaction and the detection of psychiatric morbidity in general practice. *Fam Pract* 1992;9:76–81.

Melle I, Larsen TK, Haahr U, Friis S, Johannessen JO, Opjordsmoen S, Simonsen E, Rund BR, Vaglum P, McGlashan T. Reducing the duration of untreated firstepisode psychosis: Effects on clinical presentation. *Arch Gen Psychiatry* 2004;61:143–150.

Merinder L-B. Patient education in schizophrenia: A review. *Acta Psychiatr Scand* 2000;102:98–106.

Mulvany F, O'Callaghan E, Takei N, Byrne M, Fearon P, Larkin C. Effect of social class at birth on risk and presentation of schizophrenia: Case-control study. *BMJ* 2001;323:1398–1401.

Norris FH, Kaniasty K. Received and perceived social support in times of stress: A test of the social support deterioration deterrence model. *J Pers Soc Psychol* 1996;71:498–511.

Nutt DJ, Baldwin DS, Clayton AH, Elgie R, Lecrubier Y, Montejo AL, Papakostas GI, Souery D, Trivedi MH, Tylee A. Consensus statement and research needs: The role of dopamine and norepinephrine in depression and antidepressant treatment. *J Clin Psychiatry* 2006; 67 Suppl 6:46–49.

Oliver MI, Pearson N, Coe N, Gunnell D. Help-seeking behaviour in men and women with common mental health problems: Cross-sectional study. *Br J Psychiatry* 2005;186:297–301.

Olstad R, Sexton H, Sogaard AJ. The Finnmark Study. A prospective population study of the social support buffer hypothesis, specific stressors and mental distress. *Soc Psychiatry Psychiatr Epidemiol* 2001;36:582–589.

Piccinelli M, Bisoffi G, Bon MG, Cunico L, Tansella M. Validity and test-retest reliability of the Italian version of the 12-item General Health

Questionnaire in general practice: A comparison between three scoring methods. *Compr Psychiatry* 1993;34:198–205.

Ponizovsky AM, Geraisy N, Shoshan E, Kremer I, Smetannikov E. Treatment lag on the way to the mental health clinic among Arab- and Jewish-Israeli patients. *Isr J Psychiatry Relat Sci* 2007a;44:234-243.

Ponizovsky AM, Geraisy N, Shoshan E, Kremer I, Smetannikov E, Grinshpoon A. Emotional distress among first-time patients attending outpatient mental health clinics in Israel: an Arab-Jewish comparative study. *Isr J Psychiatry Relat Sci* 2007b;44:62-70.

Rabin S, Kahan E, Zalewsky S, Rabin B, Herz M, Mehudar O, Kitai E. Primary care physicians' attitudes to battered women and feelings of self-competence regarding their care. *Isr Med Assoc J* 2000;2:753–757.

Regehr C, Hemsworth D, Hill J. Individual predictors of posttraumatic distress: A structural equation model. *Can J Psychiatry* 2001;46:156–161.

Ritsner M, Modai I, Endicott J, Rivkin O, Nechamkin Y, Barak P, Goldin V, Ponizovsky A. Differences in quality of life domains and psychopathologic and psychosocial factors in psychiatric patients. *J Clin Psychiatry* 2000;61:880–889.

Robins L N,Wing J,Wittchen HU, Helzer JE, Babor TF, Burke J, Farmer A, Jablenski A, Pickens R, Regier DA, et al. The Composite International Diagnostic Interview. An epidemiologic instrument suitable for use in conjunction with different diagnostic systems and in different cultures. *Arch Gen Psychiatry* 1988;45:1069–1077.

Sagiv L, Schwartz S. Determinants of readiness for outgroup social contact: Dominance relations and minority group motivations. *Int J Psychol* 1998;33:313–324.

Salari S. Invisible in aging research: Arab Americans,Middle Eastern immigrants, and Muslims in the United States. *Gerontologist* 2002;42:580–588.

Schwarzer R, Jerusalem M. Generalized Self-Efficacy scale. In: Weinman J, Wright S, Johnston M, editors. *Measures in health psychology: A user's portfolio. Causal and control beliefs.*Windsor, U.K.: NFER-NELSON, 1995, pp. 35–37.

Seedat S, Stein DJ, Berk M, Wilson Z. Barriers to treatment among members of a mental health advocacy group in South Africa. *Soc Psychiatry Psychiatr Epidemiol* 2002;37:483–487.

Shemesh AA, Kohn R, Blumstein T, Geraisy N, Novikov I, Levav I. A community study on emotional distress among Arab and Jewish Israelis over the age of 60. *Int J Geriatr Psychiatry* 2006;21:64–76.

Shields M. Stress, health and the benefit of social support. *Health Rep* 2004;15:9–38.

Sirey JA. Perceived stigma and patient-rated severity of illness as predictors of antidepressant drug adherence. *Psychiatr Serv* 2001;52:1615–1620.

Skaret E, Kvale G, RaadalM. General self-efficacy, dental anxiety and multiple fears among 20-year-olds in Norway. *Scand J Psychol* 2003;44:331–337.

Thoits PA. Stress, coping, and social support processes: Where are we? What next? *J Health Soc Behav* 1995;Spec No:53–79.

Turner RJ, AvisonWR. Status variations in stress exposure: Implications for the interpretation of research on race, socioeconomic status, and gender. *J Health Soc Behav* 2003;44:488–505.

Turner RJ, Marino F. Social support and social structure: A descriptive epidemiology. *J Health Soc Behav* 1994;35:193–212.

Ustun TB, Sartorius N. Public health aspects of anxiety and depressive disorders. *Int Clin Psychopharmacol* 1993; Suppl 1:15–20.

Wang PS, Berglund PA, Olfson M, Kessler RC. Delays in initial treatment contact after first onset of a mental disorder. *Health Serv Res* 2004;39:393–415.

Wang PS, Demler O, Kessler RS.Adequacy of treatment for serious mental diseases in the United States. *Am J Public Health* 2002;92:92–98.

Wells KB, BurnamMA, Camp P. Severity of depression and fee-for-service general medical and mental health specialty practices. *Med Care* 1995; 33: 350–364.

Wittchen HU, Robins LN, Cottler LB, Sartorius N, Burke JD, Regier D. Cross-cultural feasibility, reliability and sources of variance of the Composite International Diagnostic Interview (CIDI). The Multicentre WHO/ADAMHA Field Trials. *Br J Psychiatry* 1991;159:645–653.

Wu AM, Tang CS, Kwok TC. Self-efficacy, health locus of control, and psychological distress in elderly Chinese women with chronic illnesses. *Aging Ment Health* 2004;8:21–28.

Zimet GD, Dahlem NW, Zimet SG, Farley GK. The Multidimensional Scale of Perceived Social Support. *J Pers Assess* 1988;52:30–41.

Chapter 8

HEALTH SERVICE NEEDS
UNDER TERRORISM

ABSTRACT

In this chapter we describe needs for general health and mental health services among people exposed ongoing threats of war and terroristic attacks. The impact of the exposure to terrorism and psychological distress on primary care attendees in Jerusalem neighborhoods that were exposed to fire from Palestinian territories and the effects of escalation of terrorism on help-seeking in Jerusalem, a city with adequate supply of medical and psychiatric services will be discussed.

Terrorism aims to spread fear and chaos, and to create instability and distress, thereby violating the routine of daily life, and changing routines and habits of the general population (Fullerton et al., 2003). Research findings have shown that in addition to the direct victims of terror attacks, posttraumatic stress disorder symptoms have also been documented among individuals indirectly exposed to the violence. While the effects of specific mass trauma events such as the 9/11 attacks have been the focus of extensive research, the literature on the impact of ongoing exposure to terrorism is scant. Civilians exposed to severe and ongoing war trauma and terrorism are at increased risk for a host of negative post-exposure outcomes. In contrast, brief and indirect exposure usually entails only limited risk, if any, of long-term mental health problems among the general population (Weinberg et al., 2012).

The Israeli population has been subjected to the stresses of war and terrorist attacks since long before modern Israel reached independence in

1948. Jerusalem has been subjected to numerous terrorist attacks over the last 60 years (Levav et al., 2006).

From 1967 through September 2003, there were 486 attacks, with 510 persons killed and 2,636 injured (Human Rights Watch, 2002; Ministry of Foreign Affairs, 2004). During the armed Intifada (Arabic for uprising; the Palestinian uprising against Israeli occupation of the West Bank and Gaza Strip, beginning in 1987), terrorism escalated in both magnitude and lethality. Since September 2000, 1,238 people have been killed by Palestinian violence and terrorism. From 2001 through 2007, 8.342 Israelis were wounded in terror attacks (Israel Ministry of Foreign Affairs, 2013).

Israel's small size and close-knit social structure gave rise to the Israeli experience of a feeling of deep involvement with every terror attack (Bleich et al., 2003). More recently, chemical, biological, radiological, and nuclear terrorism have become an immediate threat for the world community and is particularly acute in Israel. The psychological damage and demoralization caused by the threat of terrorism can be more significant than their potential for mass destruction (DiGiovanni, 2001; Kutz and Bleich, 2003). Gelkopf et al (2013) concluded that continuous exposure to terror has a strong negative impact on mental health. However, even within a chronic situation of terror, individuals with high posttraumatic symptomatology recover over time, and though prolonged exposure to terror might exacerbate symptomatology, it does not necessarily trigger new cases of PTSD (Gelkopf et al., 2013). The very knowledge that a terrorist organization such as Hizballah or al-Qaeda had achieved nuclear capability, or was in the process of doing so, would have a severe impact on the Israeli public and on Israel's national resilience, even in the absence of an overt threat (Freilich, 2010).

Chemical or biological terror may cause mass casualties, but the major damage of such a threat centers on psychological terror (Kutz and Bleich, 2003). Decisions made and actions taken by crisis and consequence managers during the initial stages of a domestic terrorist incident that involves a weapon of mass destruction will influence the ultimate psychological toll of the disaster. Training exercises that force decision makers to confront the consequences of their decisions on the behaviors of a population at risk from a weapon of mass destruction agent release, and critically examining the capabilities of mental health crisis intervention teams that might respond to a terrorist event help crisis managers prepare for their roles (DiGiovanni, 2001).

Anxiety and panic associated with the threat of unconventional warheads can potentially disrupt lives, affect entire populations and substantially increase the demands on medical systems. In the event of an actual attack, the capacity of the hospitals to function becomes crucial. Following terror attacks, and/or the threat of chemical or biological threat or attack, the psychiatrists' role focuses on treating casualties of stress and anxiety. Psychiatrists must also be aware of the possibility that psychological and behavioral symptoms may reflect organic brain damage from pathogenic agents, and that an appropriate differential diagnosis may be life saving for the patient (Kutz and Bleich, 2003).

To examine the impact of terror attacks on the psychological well-being, our group performed a study (Yagur et al., 2002) among residents of Gilo, a Jerusalem neighborhood, that was exposed to gunfire attacks during the protracted undeclared war of the Palestinian Authority against the Israeli civilian population and that had become a threatening experience for the residents. We assessed the level of psychological distress in patients that experienced long-term exposure to gunfire, and that attended a primary care clinic in Gilo. A self-administered questionnaire exploring emotional distress (anxiety and depression symptoms), gunfire exposure, patterns of help-seeking behavior, and prescription of sedative or hypnotic drugs was administered to 125 consecutive patients who saw a general practitioner during a 10 week period in the autumn of 2001. Eighty-four patients that reside in Gilo were compared with 41 patients that reside in neighborhoods that were not under fire. Study participants were asked to answer the question "How much discomfort has the problem caused you during the past month?" in relation to nine symptoms of depression (low mood, hopelessness, helplessness, worthlessness, self-dislike, feelings of loneliness and guilt, concentration difficulties, and loss of appetite) and eight symptoms of anxiety (fear or panic attacks, feeling of tension or irritability, dread, restlessness, cold sweat, and headaches). Responses were scored on a 0–4 point frequency scale ("never" to "very often"), with higher scores indicating greater intensity of distress. Gilo residents had a significantly higher mean distress score than their counterparts in other neighborhoods ($1.1 + 0.8$ vs. $0.8 + 0.5$, $t = 1.73$, $p<0.01$); 15.5% of the former reported probable clinically significant distress. Emotional distress was associated with periods of intensive gunfire exposure, psychological care-seeking behavior, and the prescription of sedative or hypnotic drugs. The authors concluded that war-related life events seem to be associated with increased emotional distress. A motivated primary care physician could easily and reliably ascertain the patients' psychological status and identify those in need of psychological support.

To effectively treat trauma victims in the face of ongoing terrorism in Israel, it was suggested that stress casualties be referred from the emergency room, and treated by a mental health team, at a specifically designated "center for stress casualties". In addition, psychiatrists should be available for consultation with the medical teams, or to directly intervene with combined casualties in other hospital departments. At the regional or community level, multi-disciplinary mental health teams should be prepared, in existing installations designed for screening, treatment, and temporary containment of casualties. Local authorities should be responsible for the preparations and activation of the emergency services. A planned and rational usage of the media could have a critical influence on the ability of the authorities to manage the crisis situation and to shape the behavior of the population. In certain cases, the media might serve a crucial role in relaying re-assurance and instructions to citizens isolated in their homes. (Kutz and Bleich, 2003)

The Mental Health Services of the Israel Ministry of Health indeed designed and implemented a comprehensive emergency response system in general hospitals and community settings to meet the psychological needs of the community in general and of individuals in particular, following ongoing exposure to terror. The Director of Mental Health Services in the Ministry of Health and the Head of the Stress Unit serve as national coordinators of treatment for psychological trauma. District Psychiatrists are responsible for community based mental health services, and together with the District Physicians, they head the District Health Bureaus. District Psychiatrists are authorized to activate all professional mental health care resources to treat psychological trauma in emergency situations (Ministry of Health, Mental Health Services, 2003a).

During the intifada or periods of intense and frequent terror attacks the numbers of psychologically traumatized terror victims climbed steadily; the ratio of patients admitted to emergency rooms and who were psychologically traumatized to those physically traumatized by suicide bombings increased from 4:1 to 20:1 (Ben Gershon et al., 2005). A unique mental health support system was developed to avoid or ameliorate the development of psychiatric disability. Teams included a senior psychiatrist (team leader), two additional psychiatrists, two clinical psychologists, two clinical social workers, and two psychiatric nurses. Immediately following an attack, the team arrived at the emergency room of the relevant hospital to examine the casualties. After receiving first aid, patients suffering from anxiety and panic attacks were brought to the designated Stress Unit (SU) that was completely separated from the emergency room, in order to prevent secondary trauma from witnessing the treatment of severely injured victims. All individual and group interventions were performed in the SU. All patients in the stress unit were examined by a mental health professional prior to discharge. In addition to emergency supportive care, interventions in general hospitals included culturally sensitive written information in the native language of the patients (Hebrew, English, Russian, Arabic, and Amharic) about the nature of traumatic symptoms, coping methods and contact information for local mental health caregivers. This specialized team also provided emotional support for doctors and personnel that treated terror victims who were severely injured and different from the patients they routinely treated. The social workers were the liaison between the victims and family members and, helped them cope with stress and grief. They also accompanied family members to the hospital morgue when it became necessary to identify loved ones. When team members encountered patients at high risk for Acute Stress Disorder, they referred them to outpatient mental health clinics for continued treatment. Follow-up procedures were established for patients discharged to the community (Ben Gershon et al., 2005).

In addition, there are crisis hotlines such as, ERAN, Israeli Association for Emotional First Aid by Telephone. ERAN operates Israel's National Crisis Intervention Hotline, providing an anonymous and confidential service, round the clock, seven days a week, 52 weeks of the year. ERAN provides unconditional and non-judgmental emotional support for all residents of Israel including children and youth, soldiers and the elderly; in, Hebrew, Arabic and Russian.

NATAL, Israel's Trauma Center for Victims of Terror and War is another option. NATAL operates a Hot Line for immediate treatment by telephone and/or Internet and provides individual, couple and family therapy, as well as group and social care through the Social Rehabilitation Club. The process of intake and treatment begins with an initial evaluation that includes questionnaires for checking the patient's condition. If the decision is made that treatment is necessary, the clinical manager will decide what type of treatment is appropriate for the particular person and identify the appropriate caregiver. In practice, treatment takes place either in NATAL's clinic or in another location, closer to the patient's home. In most cases, treatment at NATAL combines advanced techniques for dealing with the patient's current trauma or loss, while also relating to experiences of trauma and loss, in his past and during various development stages.

Community-based surveys on the effects of terrorism emphasize adverse psychopathological effects (Bleich et al., 2003; De Lisi et al., 2003). However the findings from our data and previous service-based inquiries (Weizman et al., 1994; Nakar et al., 1996) seem contradictory. Druss and Marcus (2004) found that although in New York City, there was a statistically significant but modest increase in the proportion of individuals who had dose increases in their psychotropic medication, for most Americans, the distress associated with the September 11 attacks was not accompanied by a commensurate increase in the use of psychotropic medications. Though treatment gaps measured by true prevalence studies and services utilization rates are not new (Kohn et al., 2004), in response to terrorism, the psychiatric treatment gap is surprising. Indeed, a small gap might have been expected, because the stigma of terrorism-induced mental disorders is less than that associated with other mental disorders, and because terrorism-induced psychopathology is generally sudden and obvious compared to the gradual and unclear onset of most mental disorders. In addition, the public mental health information constantly advertised on the media during the intifada may have impacted the applications for mental health care. This apparent paradox might be explained by the fact that most trauma victims believe that their condition is a normal psychological reaction and they do not believe that psychiatric services will provide necessary relief. As Druss and Marcus (2004) stated, "In the aftermath of terrorist attacks, many Americans might have regarded their distress as a "normal" reaction... rather than as a disorder needing (psychiatric) care...". Strous (2013) noted that many would argue that the focal point of mental health professionals during times of conflict should be swayed to focus on resilience rather than on pathology. Thus it is expected that the diminishing of stress after trauma is normal. In this age of an increasing culture of trauma, and extension of the boundaries of psychiatric injury during times of conflict, psychiatrists have an ethical responsibility to ensure that trauma and its effects during conflict are placed in its appropriate context, and that pathological responses should not received disproportionate attention (Strous, 2013).

In addition, epidemiological studies might exaggerate the scope of trauma-related psychopathology (Bleich et al., 2003; DeLisi et al., 2003); up to 14.3% of those living in close proximity to the World Trade Center in Manhattan surveyed in October 2001 met criteria for PTSD or depression (Galea et al., 2004). In contrast with these results, Northern Ireland psychiatrists stated: "because someone experiences or witnesses an act of violence does not mean that . . . (he or she) will inevitably develop psychiatric morbidity" (de Jong, et al., 2001). Somer (2008) found that considering the nature and length of the Israeli traumatic experience, the psychological impact may be considered moderate, which may result from a habituation process to the ongoing terror attacks, and to coping mechanisms.

A study was undertaken during the Al-Aqsa intifada (Levav et al., 2006) to explore the effects of the escalation of terrorism on the help-seeking behavior of the general population in Jerusalem, i.e., on its needs for medical and psychiatric services. Using time-series analyses, the authors compared the utilization of different health services, such as primary medical care and ambulance calls, and mental health services, such as psychiatric clinics, hospitals, and telephone hotlines, by Jerusalem residents before and during the intifada. The authors evaluated seasonality, general linear trends, short-term intifada impact (reflecting reactions that peaked at the third month and ended 1 year thereafter), and long-term impact (starting at the intifada outbreak and reflecting a more stable population behavior). Findings from the study did not reveal any changes in the rate of adult psychiatric outpatient visits. The elderly population, however, had both short- and long-term increases in the number of visits for their ongoing care. The proportion of recorded ICD-10 diagnoses reflecting intifada-related reactions remained generally stable. Short-term effects included an increase in psychiatric readmissions. First contacts to substance abuse clinics remained unchanged. While long-term effects included a decrease in new psychiatric hospitalizations, the rate of monthly visits to general practitioners and the number of monthly ambulance and hotline calls increased. Thus, except for the elderly and previously hospitalized persons, Jerusalem residents did not increase their use of psychiatric services but did increase their use of some other health services. These results suggest that this terrorism-affected population did not perceive their mental and social suffering as requiring specialized intervention.

The Israeli case demonstrates both the extensive effects of repeated terrorist attacks and their limitations. While Israelis were seriously affected by Palestinian terrorist attacks, this did not result in major, lasting changes in Israeli behavior. Despite being profoundly affected by terrorism, Israeli society was not demoralized by it. This is because the Israeli public grew accustomed to chronic terrorism and possessed a high level of social resilience (Waxman, 2011).

In order to benefit from psychiatric services, one must be aware of the dangers of succumbing to distress, and appropriate effect care must be available. The mental health component in primary health care needs to be empowered in emergencies, as recommended by the World Health Organization (Mental Health in Emergencies: Mental and Social Aspects of Populations Exposed to Extreme Stressors. Geneva, World Health Organization, 2003). Community based mental health facilities need to collaborate with general practitioners in order to deal with the spectrum of trauma-related reactions (Levav et al., 2006).

REFERENCES

Ben-Gershon B, Grinshpoon A, Ponizovsky A. Mental Health Services Preparing for the Psychological Consequences of Terrorism. *J Aggres Maltreat Trauma* 2005;10:743-753.

Bleich A, Gelkopf M, Solomon Z. Exposure to terrorism, stress-related mental health symptoms, and coping behaviors among a nationally representative sample in Israel. *J Am Med Assoc* 2003 6;290:612-620.

de Jong JTVM, Komproe IH, Van Ommeren M, El Masri M, Araya M, Khaled van de Put W, Somasundaram D. Lifetime events and posttraumatic stress disorder in four post-conflict settings. *J Am Med Assoc* 2001; 286:555–562.

DeLisi LE, Maurizio A, Yost M, Papparozzi CF, Fulchino C, Katz CL, Altesman J, Biel M, Lee J, Stevens P. A survey of New Yorkers after the Sept 11, 2001, terrorist attacks. *Am J Psychiatry* 2003;160:780–783.

DiGiovanni C. Pertinent psychological issues in the immediate management of a weapon of mass destruction event. *Mil Med* 2001;166(12 Suppl):59-60.

Druss BG, Marcus SC. Use of psychotropic medications before and after Sept 11, 2001. *Am J Psychiatry* 2004;161:1377–1383.

Fullerton, Ursano and Norwood, Terrorism and Disaster: Individual and community. *Mental Health Interventions*. Cambridge University Press, Cambridge, UK, 2003.

Freilich C. The Armageddon scenario: Israel and the threat of nuclear terrorism. In: *Midease Security and Policy Studies No. 84*. The Begin-Sadat Center for Strategic Studies, Bar Ilan University, April 2010, http://www.biu.ac.il/Besa/MSPS84.pdf (accessed 13.11.2013).

Galea S, Boscarino J, Resnick H, Vlahov, D. Mental health in New York City after the September 11 terrorist attacks: results from two population surveys, in Mental Health United States 2002. Rockville, Md, Substance Abuse and Mental Health Services Administration, 2004, pp. 89–97.

Gelkopf M, Solomon Z, Bleich A. A longitudinal study of changes in psychological responses to continuous terroris. *Isr J Psychiatry Relat Sci* 2013;50:100-109.

Human Rights Watch web site: www.hrs.org/reports/2002/isrpa

Israel Ministry of Foreign Affairs. http://www.mfa.gov.il/mfa/foreignpolicy/terrorism/palestinian/pages/ 2013.

Kohn R, Saxena S, Saraceno B, Levav I: Treatment gap in mental health care. *Bull World Health Org* 2004;82:858–866.

Kutz I, Bleich A. Conventional, chemical and biological terror of mass destruction: Psychological aspects and psychiatric guidelines. In J. Shemer & Y. Schoenfeld (Eds.), *Terror and medicine.* Lengeirich, Germany: Science Publishers, 2003, pp. 533-544.

Levav I, Novikov I, Grinshpoon A, Rosenblum J, Ponizovsky A. Health services utilization in Jerusalem under terrorism. *Am J Psychiatry* 2006;163:1355-1361.

Mental Health in Emergencies: Mental and Social Aspects of Populations Exposed to Extreme Stressors. Geneva, World Health Organization, 2003.

Nakar S, Kahan E, Nir T, Weingarten MA. The influence of SCUD missile attacks on the utilization of ambulatory services in a family practice. *Med Confl Surviv* 1996;12:149–153.

Somer E. Exposure to repeated acts of terrorism: perspectives from an attacked community Based on a paper presented at a colloquium at the Alice Salomon University of Applied Sciences, Berlin, Germany, February, 2007 Klinische Sozialarbeit 4(Sonderausgabe) 2008, pp. 6-11.

Strous R. Ethical considerations during times of conflict: Challenges and pitfalls for the psychiatrist. *Isr J Psychiatry Relat Sci* 2013;50:122-129.

Waxman D. Living with Terror, not Living in Terror: The Impact of Chronic Terrorism on Israeli Society. Perspectives on Terrorism 2011. Terrorism Research Initiative 2011;5:4-26.

Weinberg M, Besser A, Campeas M, Shvil E,Neria Y. Civilians Exposed to Terrorism and War Trauma in Israel: The Role of Intra–and Inter–Personal Factors. *Advances in Psychology Research. Volume 94* Nova Science Press, 2012. https://www.novapublishers.com/catalog/product_info.php?products_id=33577.

Weizman R, Laor N, Barber Y, Selman A, Schujovizky A, Wolmer L, Laron Z, Gil-Ad I. Impact of the Gulf War on the anxiety, cortisol, and growth hormone levels of Israeli civilians. *Am J Psychiatry* 1994;151:71–75.

Yagur A, Grinshpoon A, Ponizovsky A. Primary care clinic attenders under war stress. *Isr Med Assoc J* 2002;4:568–572.

Chapter 9

PSYCHIATRIC EMERGENCY SERVICES

ABSTRACT

This chapter describes the introduction and first-year experience of emergency psychiatric services provided via the national medical emergency service ("Magen David Adom") that serves as a screening hotline and an expert psychiatrist.

Psychiatric emergency has been defined as "an acute clinical situation in which there is imminent risk of serious harm or death to self or others unless there is some immediate intervention." (Keespies, 1998)

In contrast, a crisis has been described as "a serious disruption in the individual's baseline functioning, such that coping strategies are inadequate to restore equilibrium." (Emergency Mental Health, 2000). Crises tend to become emergencies when the patient's needs are not adequately met by the broader health and social systems.

Phelan (1996) categorized three types of psychiatric emergencies or crises:

a) Psycho-social crises among people who may not have a formal mental illness and who might not have had previous contact with mental health services

b) Recurring psycho-social crises for people with mild or moderate mental health problems, drug or alcohol problems and/or personality disorders

c) Relapse and/or social difficulties with potentially catastrophic consequences among people with psychotic disorders

Although psychiatric emergencies seem to erupt suddenly, their origins are usually nowhere near the entrance to the emergency department which is the gateway to hospitalization, the last resort in psychiatric treatment (Minghella et al., 1998).

Twenty-four -hour care is required for people in acute mental health crises (Department of Health, 1996), and it has become evident that emergency departments in general hospitals are not equipped to deal with psychiatric emergencies (Audit Commission, 1996).

Psychiatric emergencies require rapid response to urgent requests for help, preferably in the client's residence or in his own environment, in order to avoid hospitalization (Burti and Tansell, 1995). During the early 1930's, in Amsterdam, Querido established one of the earliest examples of a "psychiatric first aid service" (Querido, 1968).

Following the Great Depression of 1929, in the 1930's it was imperative to reduce the costs of care. In Amsterdam alone there were about 3000 inpatients in psychiatric hospitals. The municipality considered it worthwhile to invest in the salary of one psychiatrist in an attempt to reduce the costs of psychiatric hospitalizations. Considering that it was more efficient to avoid hospitalization rather than discharge patients, screening for all potential psychiatric admissions was requested by physicians, police or other authorities. This led to the establishment of the "psychiatric first aid service". Indeed, from the implementation of the service in 1931 until World War II, the number of patient days in mental hospitals did not increase. Although admissions, readmissions and discharges increased, the average length of stay was reduced and hospitalization became fluid. This change led to recognition of the patient as part of the community and hospital stay became merely a link in a chain of events that links society to the hospital (Querido, 1968).

MacMillan (1958) and Carse et al (1958) reported the existence of home treatment services as early as 1949 in Nottingham and Worthing in the United Kingdom, respectively, and Meyer et al (1967) described psychiatric home visits in Boston USA, beginning in 1957.

Emergency psychiatric home care has since evolved to mobile crisis units which have been broadly discussed in the literature (Robin et al., 2008; Currier et al., 2010; Murphy, 2012; Murphy et al., 2012). Mobile crisis teams have been described as 'a van staffed by health professionals, typically a psychiatrist, a social worker and a registered nurse who provide at-home crisis intervention for patients suffering psychiatric trauma' (Chiu and Primeau, 1991). However, even in multidisciplinary mobile teams, there was generally only one staff member on call during the night shift (Burti and Tansell, 1995).

Ambulatory care for individuals with severe mental disorders has been shown to be a valid alternative to hospitalization. Robin et al (2008) investigated the utility of using ambulatory care services by a mobile crisis intervention team in response to all requests for first hospitalizations in a psychiatric department. They sought to determine whether the crisis intervention team could provide an adequate alternative to inpatient care and investigated whether ambulatory care ultimately resulted in shorter or less hospitalizations. In a prospective, comparative, cohort study over a 5-year period beginning with the initiation of the ambulatory care unit in one of the hospital departments, all patients that arrived to that department for the first time were offered immediate ambulatory care for 1 month. Duration of hospital stay and number of days in hospital was compared with that of inpatients in other departments in the same hospital. Regardless of diagnosis, intensive follow-up home care, based on systemic crisis intervention was found to be an effective and well-accepted alternative to hospitalization. A highly significant immediate decrease in both the number of admissions and the duration of hospital stay was observed for the experimental group, with no subsequent increase in the number of days of hospitalization. The results support the use of ambulatory crisis intervention services from psychiatric hospitals.

In a recent Cochrane review Murphy et al (2012) revealed that crisis intervention appears to reduce repeat admissions to hospital after the initial 'index' crises. In the studies evaluated, they found that, this was particularly true for mobile crisis teams that supported patients in their own homes. Crisis intervention seemed to reduce family burden and proved to be a more satisfactory form of care for both patients and families. Three months after the index crisis, the mental state of patients treated by mobile crisis teams was superior to those who received standard care. Some studies found crisis interventions to be more cost effective than hospital care. There was no data on staff satisfaction, or number of relapses. The authors concluded that care based on crisis intervention principles, with or without an ongoing home care package, appears to be a viable and acceptable way of treating people with serious mental illnesses, however more evaluative studies are needed.

Guo et al (2001) compared emergency mobile crisis intervention and hospital based intervention cohorts, each with 1100 patients and found that patients treated via hospital based intervention was 51% more likely to be *hospitalized within one month following the crisis (p<.001). This study provides empirical evidence that mobile crisis interventions might reduce hospital admissions (Guo et al., 2000).*

In many countries, there is an emergency services phone number (e.g., 911 in the United States or 101 in Israel) that allows the caller to contact local emergency services for help. In a retrospective study, Scott (2000) evaluated the efficiency of a mobile crisis intervention program for 111 phone calls to 911 that were identified as psychiatric emergencies. 73 of the crises were handed by a mobile crisis team and 58 were handled by standard police intervention. Forty-five percent of the emergencies handled by the emergency mobile unit lead to hospitalization compared to 72% of the emergencies handled by the police. The results of this study justify introduction of mobile crisis programs as an integral component of health care, pending more rigorous evaluation of the costs and benefits of mobile crisis services (Scott, 2000).

A new integrated service of 24/7 telephone support backed by physicians and plainclothes policemen, with an ambulance when necessary was recently introduced in Canada. Similar to the pre-World War II experience in Amsterdam (Querido, 1968), in spite of increased service use, actual duration of interventions by staff members was reduced. Patients treated by the service later revealed an increase in outpatient visits (Kiseley et al., 2010).

Reding and Raphelson (1995) reported findings of retrospective study that evaluated the effect of adding a psychiatrist to a 24-hour mobile crisis intervention team, on the number of admissions, to the local state and private hospitals. During the program, the psychiatrist provided immediate psychiatric treatment on site. There was a sharp decrease in state hospital admissions and no increase in private hospital admissions when the psychiatrist was part of the mobile crises intervention team. When the psychiatrist was removed from the team there was a rebound and increase in hospital admissions.

EMERGENCY PSYCHIATRIC SERVICES IN ISRAEL

Mental Health Hotlines

ERAN (Emotional First Aid by Telephone, http://www.eran.org.il/)

ERAN operates Israel's National Crisis Intervention Hotline, which is an emotional first-aid Hotline that provides an anonymous and confidential service 24/7. ERAN volunteers are trained to provide support and empower callers to search for emotional resilience and survivability in the face of personal crises that individuals might experience. The Eran staff is comprised of over a thousand volunteers that are highly trained over a period of 12 months. In addition, ERAN volunteers often encounter suicidal callers, and they are to endeavor to recognize immediate danger, prevent the attempt and when necessary, alert emergency and welfare authorities for further direct action. On an average day there are 394 calls to Eran, 144,000 calls a year. Eran received 800 calls about suicide cases in progress, and hundreds of calls from those suffering from panic and anxiety ERAN also provides emotional Support via the Internet: Email: info@eran.org.il (Hebrew and English); Online Chat - direct access through the Hebrew website, ICQ - #12010. Services are provided in Hebrew, Arabic and Russian.

NATAL Israel Trauma Center for Victims of Terror and War (http://www.natal.org.il/English/)

Natal is an organization that provides emotional and psychological support to Israelis that suffer from Post Traumatic Stress Disorder (PTSD) as a result of the Arab-Israeli conflict. NATAL operates a toll free national hotline that is staffed by trained volunteers, and provides subsidized and even free, clinical treatment services to trauma victims and their family members. NATAL services are intended for individuals who experienced traumatic events resulting from the Arab-Israel conflict, and for members of the victims' families. Services are also available to high risk populations, i.e., residents of the confrontation line, discharged soldiers and parents of combat soldiers.

SAHAR (http://www.sahar.org.il)

SAHAR is a non-profit organization that offers emotional support via the Internet from 9:00 pm to midnight, to people in emotional distress, on the brink of suicide, or people who are considering or contemplating suicide. SAHAR uses various different web-based media (email, chat, ICQ), to offer immediate service to applicants, who may either remain anonymous or identify themselves by name. All SAHAR volunteers are trained by professionals in related fields, and have a good understanding and use of internet communication.

Psychiatric Services

In Israel, public community-based mental health services are available only during working hours. In the event of a psychiatric crisis outside of office hours, emergency rooms in general and/or psychiatric hospitals offer the only option for treatment. Transportation to emergency rooms for patients experiencing acute psychiatric crises is often problematic, and used as a last resort. When patient safety and security, or the safety of those in the patient's environment is endangered, the police are often called to intervene. This is typical of police involvement in psychiatric emergencies world over (Querido, 1968; Scott, 2000). Lacking the appropriate training the police often respond inappropriately or refuse to respond at all, on the grounds that mental illness is not a police responsibility. The staff of the Magen David Adom (MaDA), the national medical emergency service, is also not equipped or trained for emergency mental health interventions (Khwaled et al., 2009).

Home visits are sometimes requested by the District Psychiatrists, in crises situations that fall under the provisions of the Mental Patients Treatment Act, 1991. In addition, although home visits are included in the basket of services provided by outpatient clinics in the public sector of the mental health service system, staff shortages often preclude their implementation.

Abarbanel Mental Health Center in Ramat Gan, initiated a'Mobile Unit' project that was designed as an 'outreach' service, and provided home based patient care to encourage motivation for rehabilitation and avoidance of re-hospitalization. Success was immediate and substantial, however the service was available only to individuals previously diagnosed with mental disorders who were "in the system". Tirat Carmel Mental Health Center also has a home care unit, designed to treat its own discharged patients who fail to attend the outpatient clinic for follow-up care (Dr. Grinshpoon, personal communication, 2006).

The Israeli Community Emergency Psychiatric Service (CEPS) was initiated by the Mental Health Services at the Ministry of Health along with the Forensic Psychiatry Unit and was implemented in May 2005 in the Tel Aviv and Central Districts with a team of licensed psychiatrists. In addition, an emergency call center was established in the emergency room of the Beersheba Mental Health Center for the Southern District.

The launching of the pilot project was advertised in Hebrew, Arabic and Russian in the daily newspapers. In the event of psychiatric distress or emergency the public was instructed to dial 101 the emergency service phone number for Magen David Adom (MaDA) emergency care services. The

MaDA dispatchers, who determine which MaDA vehicle to dispatch, were now able to respond to calls involving psychiatric emergencies. The Ministry of Health engaged a pool of about 8 licensed psychiatrists to be available on-call one per shift. By the 25th of each month, the MaDA dispatchers were given a list prepared by the District Psychiatrist, of the names and telephone numbers of on-call psychiatrists for the following month. The dispatchers referred 'mental health' callers to the on-call psychiatrist.

Once contacted, the on call psychiatrist could either:

a. advise the caller what treatment options were available, or refer him/her to an outpatient clinic or hospital emergency room, as necessary

b. perform a home visit, including emergency administration of medication. If the patient would agree to be diagnosed and treated, the psychiatrist would give a provisional diagnosis and recommend treatment that might include a letter of referral to an appropriate facility. If the client would not consent to diagnosis and treatment the on-call psychiatrist would record the case and determine if the situation warranted contacting the District Psychiatrist to issue a Compulsory Examination Order in accord with Mental Patients Treatment Act, 1991.

Payments for the home visits were collected by the psychiatrist, except when a fee-waiver was called for. When a hospitalization order is issued, or if the visiting psychiatrist contacts the District Psychiatrist to issue a compulsory evaluation, the cost of the service is covered by the government.

In the first year activity, from May 31, 2005 to June 1, 2006, a total of 1,472 calls were made to the on-call psychiatrists, of which 198 (13.5%) resulted in a referral to ambulatory care, 116 (7.8%) resulted in a home visit, 50 (3.4%) resulted (after the psychiatrist's examination) in voluntary hospitalization and 16 (1.1%) resulted in compulsory hospitalization.

In addition, the following patient group profile was outlined based on the analysis of 97 calls (August, 1996): female, age 19-35, unmarried, diagnosis - schizophrenia, no previous psychiatric hospitalizations, presenting no danger to herself or others. The majority of the applications to the emergency service came from family members (61.2%). The vast majority of the calls (90%) did not require a home visit and a recommendation for ambulatory care was considered sufficient for 37.3% of the patients. Only 14.9% were referred to inpatient care and in most of these cases hospitalization was voluntary. When there was no home visit, the psychiatrist followed the case until the client received the recommended care. Ten percent of the calls that required home visits entailed a preliminary diagnosis of psychosis and the need for crisis intervention or administration of psychotropic medication.

Although, consistent with previous studies (Bebbington et al., 1994), most calls for intervention in this project concerned persons with schizophrenia or who were in a psychotic state which is a major risk factor for violent behavior (Reicher and Rossler, 1991), only 20% of the cases were assessed by the psychiatrist as danger to self or others and only 1% were hospitalized involuntarily. These figures contrast to the ad-hoc reservations expressed by some of the participating psychiatrists concerning performing home visits unescorted, or apprehension regarding the ability to cope with a range of pathologies and medical needs without the backup of an expert support system. Noteworthy, only eight psychiatrists agreed to join the project and within a month four of these had dropped out.

A joint draft of procedures was drawn up by the Ministry of Health, Magen David Adom and the Israel Police Force. The declared purpose of the procedures was to delineate the required response to psychiatric emergencies in order to provide appropriate quick response in the to the person in need of help while protecting patient's rights and dignity as well as public safety. The procedures focus on psychiatric emergencies that involve criminal behavior of individuals with suspected mental disorders. Responsibility for implementation of the procedures rests with the District Psychiatrist, Israel Police Department and Magen David Adom. The basis for the procedures includes The Law for the Treatment of the Mentally Ill (1991), Regulations for the Treatment of the Mentally Ill, 1992, Basic Law for Human Dignity and Libergy, 1992, Law of Patient's Rights, 1996, Criminal Procedure (Enforcement Powers - Arrests) Law 1996. In accord with the procedures, if the police officer determines that an individual requires an emergency psychiatric evaluation, such as in the case of a suicidal threat, and if the individual refuses to go to a psychiatric emergency room with the police officer, and the police officer thinks that a psychiatric evaluation is necessary to protect the patient or the patient's environment, the policeman must report to the commanding officer or medical authority in the station who will in turn refer to the District Psychiatrist to receive instructions as to how to proceed. The District Psychiatrist can then instruct the police to bring the individual to an emergency room, and the District Psychiatrist would then issue an order for a compulsory psychiatric evaluation

(Ministry of Health, Magen David Adom, Israel Police Force, Procedure 75.007, August 2005).

Given that the responsibility for mental health care was transferred from the Ministry of Health to the health maintenance organizations (HMOs), the community emergency service service should have been adjusted to the needs of the HMOs. This unique but necessary service was not provided by the network of public sector mental health services, however despite our successful experience it was discontinued in March 2013 as it was not included in the national basket of mental health services.

CONCLUSION

We suggest that CEPS should be reconsidered, as it might play a preventive role by enabling the early detection of mental illness, preventing deterioration and consequent hospitalization. In the case of pre-existing mental disorders, CEPS raises the awareness of mental disorders and offers family members an opportunity to encourage patients to improve cooperation with available services and treatment.

Community psychiatry involves reaching out into the community and to provide flexible services which meet the various needs of individuals with mental disorders. Provision of early intervention in emergency situations clearly remains a difficult and complex task (Katching, 1995).

REFERENCES

Audit Commission By Accident or Design 1996 Audit Commission *By Accident or Design*. HMSO: London, 1996.

Bebbington PE, Feeney ST, Flannigan CB, Lack S, Birkett P, Lynch S, Johnson T. Inner London collaborative audit of admissions in two health districts II: Ethnicity and the use of the Mental Health Act. *Br J Psychiatry* 1994;165:743–749.

Burti L, Tansella M. Acute home-based care and community psychiatry In: Phelan M, Stratahdee G, Thornicroft G (Eds.). *Emergency Mental health Services in the Community*. Cambridge University Press: Cambridge, 1995, pp. 276-298.

Carse J, Panton NE, Watt A. A District Mental Health Service: the Worthing experiment. *Lancet* 1958;1(7010):39-41.

Chiu TL, Primeau C. A psychiatric mobile crisis unit in New York City: description and assessment, with implications for mental health care in the 1990s. *Int J Soc Psychiatry* 1991;37:251-258.

Currier GW, Fisher SG, Caine ED. Mobile crisis team intervention to enhance linkage of discharged suicidal emergency department patients to outpatient psychiatric services: a randomized controlled trial. *Acad Emerg Med* 2010;17:36-43.

Department of Health. *The Spectrum of Care: local services for people with mental health problems.* HMSO: London, 1996.

Emergency mental health: Educational manual,2000,. p. 14. Available at: http://www.mheccu.ubc.ca/documents/publications/emh-manual.pdf

Guo S, Biegel DE, Johnsen JA, Dyches H. Assessing the impact of community-based mobile crisis services on preventing hospitalization. *Psychiatr Serv* 2001;52:223-228.

Katching H. The scope and limitations of emergency mental health services in the community. In: Michael Phelan, Geraldine Stradhdee, Graham Thornicroft. *Emergency mental health services in the community.* Cambridge University Press, Cambridge, 1995.

Khawaled R, Bauer A, Rosca P, Helman D, Shai U, Grinshpoon A, Ponizovsky AM. Community emergency psychiatric service in Israel: a one-year experience. *Isr J Psychiatry Relat Sci* 2009;46:207-212.

Kisely S, Campbell LA, Peddle S, Hare S, Pyche M, Spicer D, Moore B. A controlled before-and-after evaluation of a mobile crisis partnership between mental health and police services in Nova Scotia. *Can J Psychiatry* 2010;55:662-668.

Kleespies, P.M. (Ed.). *Emergencies in mental health practice: Evaluation and management.* New York: Guilford Press, 1998.

Macmillan D. Community treatment of mental illness. *Lancet* 1958;2(7039):201-204.

Meyer RE, Schiff LF, Becker A. The home treatment of psychotic patients: an analysis of 154 cases. *Am J Psychiatry* 1967;123:1430-1438.

Minghella E., Ford R., Freeman T, Hoult J, McGlynn P, O'Halloran P. Open all hours: 24 hour response for people with mental health emergencies. *Salisbury Centre for Mental Health*, London, 1998.

Ministry of Health, Magen David Adom, Israel Police Force, Procedure 75.007, August 2005, prepared by Kwaled R, Bauer A, Kalian M, approved by Grinshpoon A, Feigenberg Z, and Belcher A.

Murphy K. Crisis intervention teams and mobile crisis management. *N C Med J* 2012;73:200.

Murphy S, Irving CB, Adams CE, Driver R. Crisis intervention for people with severe mental illnesses. *Cochrane Database Syst Rev* 2012;5:CD001087.

Phelan M. Models of crisis intervention. In: *Effectively managing mental health service development.* Thompson K. and Strathdee G. (Eds). Sainsbury Centre for Mental Health: London, 1996.

Querido, A. The shaping of community mental health care. *Br J Psychiatry* 1968;114:293-302.

Reding GR, Raphelson M. Around-the-clock mobile psychiatric crisis intervention: another effective alternative to psychiatric hospitalization. *Community Ment Health J* 1995;31:179-187.

Riecher A, Rossler W, Loffler W. Factors influencing compulsory admission of psychiatric patients. *Psychol Med* 1991;21:197–201.

Robin M, Bronchard M, Kannas S. Ambulatory care provision versus first admission to psychiatric hospital: 5 years follow up. *Soc Psychiatry Psychiatr Epidemiol* 2008;43:498-506.

Scott RL. Evaluation of a mobile crisis program: effectiveness, efficiency, and consumer satisfaction. *Psychiatr Serv* 2000;51:1153-1156.

Chapter 10

ORAL HEALTH NEEDS OF PATIENTS WITH MENTAL ILLNESS

ABSTRACT

People with severe mental illness tend to be more susceptible to oral disease because of poor oral hygiene, fear, specific dental phobias, dental costs, difficulty in accessing healthcare facilities, hesitancy of some dentists to treat special populations, and the side-effects of psychiatric drugs such as dry mouth. In this chapter the reasons for poor oral health among individuals with severe mental disorders are presented, together with descriptions of methods for evaluating oral dental status and proposed solutions for improving dental care and thus quality of life of this population, whether in the community or within the hospital. The impact of dental services for psychiatric inpatients and outpatients implemented in accord with the mental health reform in Israel is described in detail.

IMPORTANCE OF ORAL HEALTH

In addition to affecting how we eat, chew and taste food, oral health has psychological impact on self-esteem and quality of life by influencing how we look, speak, socialize and enjoy life (Kisely et al., 2011; Jyoti et al., 2012, Shah et al., 2012). Oral health is an important component of general physical health. Poor oral health has been linked to systemic diseases such as coronary heart disease, stroke and respiratory disease (Kisely et al., 2011) Recently, it has been recognized that oral infection, especially periodontitis, may affect the course and pathogenesis of a number of systemic diseases, such as cardiovascular disease, bacterial pneumonia and diabetes mellitus (Li et al., 2000). In addition, second generation antipsychotic agents have been associated with an increase in metabolic disorders such as diabetes, which may compound the problem.

REASONS FOR POOR ORAL HEALTH AMONG PSYCHIATRIC PATIENTS

People with severe mental illness often have advanced oral diseases because psychiatric disorders often entail changes in behavior, neglect of social contacts, loss of concern for general and oral health, and decline or total neglect of oral hygiene (Jovanavic et al., 2010). People with severe mental illness tend to be more susceptible to oral disease because of poor oral hygiene, fear, specific dental phobias, dental costs, difficulty in accessing healthcare facilities and the side-effects of psychiatric drugs (Barlow et al., 2001; Ramon et al., 2003). In the context of mental health, dental care has low priority and in some phases of illness, does not exist. Many psychiatric patients do not regularly visit a dentist or brush their teeth. Many psychiatric patients are not even aware of the need for dental care. The apathy of caregivers and the staff and administrators of long-term facilities and the inaccessibility of dental services aggravate existing dental problems. (Jyoti et al., 2012).

In addition, long term treatment with antipsychotic agents might have adverse effects on oral health by increasing the risk for oral diseases and their duration. For patients treated with psychotropic drugs, the most frequently encountered adverse effect of dental importance is xerostomia (dry mouth). The patient feels dryness in the mouth, and the lack of saliva can lead to dental caries and candidosis (Javonovic et al., 2010). Individuals with schizophrenia also have an increased propensity to develop adverse orofacial effects such as sialorrhea and oral dyskinesia caused by psychotropic medications. (Friedlander and Marder, 2002; Friedlander and Liberman, 1991). Most antidepressant agents can cause xerostomia. Anticholinergic medications, such as the tricyclic antidepressants are more likely to lead to oral complications because of its prolonged effects on salivary function. Newer antidepressants such as venlafaxine, reboxetine and the selective serotonin reuptake inhibitors

(SSRIs) as well as psychostimulants can cause mild and transient dry mouth (Page, 2007).

Grinshpoon et al (2014) performed a cross-sectional study to examine the association between dental conditions in hospitalized schizophrenia patients and type of antipsychotic medication they received. Based on the literature suggesting that atypical antipsychotics (atypicals) are considered more tolerable than typical antipsychotics (Tani et al., 2012), and hypothesized that hospitalized schizophrenia patients treated with atypical antipsychotics would have better dental health than (a) those treated with typical antipsychotics and (b) those treated with a combination of both types of antipsychotics.

As hypothesized, patients treated with atypicals had better dental health than those who received typicals but not those treated with a combination of both types of antipsychotics. The atypicals group's overall decay level was significantly lower compared to the typicals group, indicating that patients maintained on atypicals have significantly more treated (filled) teeth and significantly less extracted (missing) teeth. The results of the mixed treatment group (atypicals combined with typicals) fell in between the atypicals and typicals groups in all measures.

Poor oral health has long been documented among institutionalized individuals (Ramon et al., 2003). Research worldwide has shown that this vulnerable population has more extracted or carious teeth, fewer filled teeth, more advanced periodontal disease, poorer oral hygiene, and more frequent xerostomia than the general population (Ramon et al., 2003; McCreadie et al., 2004; Jovanovic et al., 2010). The higher rate of missing teeth among psychiatric patients suggests that although dental implants have become the standard of care in the general population, it is questionable whether psychiatric patients generally benefit from that standard of treatment.

Janardhanan et al (2011) reported that people with schizophrenia tend to receive suboptimal oral health care. They might be more prone to developing dental disease because of their impaired ability to plan; their lack of motivation; and difficulty performing oral hygiene procedures. People with schizophrenia face additional obstacles because of some dentists' reluctance to treat people with symptoms of severe mental illness (Janardhanan et al., 2011).

MEASURING DENTITION

DMFT (decayed missed filled teeth) and DMFS (decayed, missing and filled surfaces) describe the prevalence of dental caries in an individual.

DMFT and DMFS are means to numerically express the caries prevalence and are obtained by calculating the number of Decayed (D) Missing (M) and Filled (F) teeth (T) or surfaces (S).

It is calculated either for 28 (permanent) teeth, excluding 18, 28, 38 and 48 (the "wisdom" teeth) or for 32 teeth (The Third edition of "Oral Health Surveys - Basic methods", Geneva 1987, recommends 32 teeth). How many teeth have caries lesions? How many teeth have been extracted? How many teeth have fillings or crowns? The sum of the three figures forms the DMFT-value. For example: DMFT of 4-3-9=16 means that 4 teeth are decayed, 3 teeth are missing and 9 teeth have fillings. It also means that 12 teeth are intact (Oral Health Database: http://www.mah.se/CAPP/Methods-and-Indices/for-Caries-prevalence/).

In a systematic review and meta-analysis of studies from the past 20 years evaluating advanced dental disease in people with severe mental illness, Kisely et al (2011) assessed the total tooth loss (edentulousness), the end-stage of both untreated caries and periodontal disease and dental decay through standardized measures: the mean number of decayed, missing and filled teeth (DMFT) or surfaces (DMFS). Nine studies were included in their meta-analysis. They found that psychiatric patients ($n = 1622$) had over three times the odds of having lost all their teeth (95% CI 1.6-7.2) compared with controls ($n = 22\ 448$). In a survey performed in the United Kingdom, most patients reported that neither the hospital staff nor caregivers in the community had ever asked them about any dental problems.

In a cross-sectional study of 133 patients attending the psychiatric outpatient department compared to 133 patients attending the general outpatient department Shah et al (2012) conducted a study to assess the oral health of psychiatric patients of Jamnagar City in the Indian state of Gujarat. The prevalence of dental caries was found to be 54.89%. Mean decayed missed filled teeth (DMFT) and decayed, missing and filled surfaces (DMFS) scores for the study group were 2.10±1.7 and 3.07±3.9 compared to 1.36±1.9 and 2.03±4.5 in the control group. Studies conducted by Tang et al (2004) in Hong-Kong reported a higher prevalence, with a mean DMFT score of 9.5±8.9. Other studies of dental care conducted among psychiatric patients also reported higher prevalence rates. Mirza et al (2001) reported a prevalence of 65.5%, Ramon et al (2003) reported a mean DMFT of 26.74, Angellillo et al (1995) reported 15.5 and Rekha et al (2002) reported 6.1. Shukla and Shrivastava (1983) in their "A psychiatric study of cases attending the dental OPD of a teaching general hospital in Jhansi" reported a lower prevalence rate of 28%. Kumar et al (2006) reported caries prevalence rate of 32.2% with mean DMFT and DMFS scores of 0.92±1.8 and 2.54±5.0. The lower prevalence rate in the Jamnagar City study may be explained by a higher concentration of fluoride in water in Jamnagar city. Moreover DMFT and DMFS scores increased with age; these findings are similar with the findings of other studies (Tang et al., 2004; Ramon et al., 2003), although the difference was not statistically significant. The mean Oral Hygiene Index – simplex (OHI-S) was 3.6±1.0 for study group and 1.2±0.9 for the control group. As the age increased, the oral health status in terms of OHI-S worsened supporting findings of previous studies (Mirza et al., 2001; Angelillo et al., 1995).

To determine oral health status and identify predictors of oral health in a representative sample of psychiatric in-patients in Serbia, Jovanovic et al (2010) performed a study that included 186 psychiatric in-patients and 186 control participants without psychiatric illness matched to the study group by age, sex, marital status, education level, employment, and monthly income. The DMFT index; community periodontal index; and plaque indexes were calculated for all participants. Interviews about their dental health behavior were conducted and medical records of all participants were examined. Psychiatric in-patients had more caries, poorer periodontal health, and poorer oral hygiene than controls. The average DMFT score for patients was 24.4 compared to 16.1 for controls ($p<0.001$). Periodontal diseases were significantly more prevalent among psychiatric in-patients than among controls ($p<0.001$). The average plaque index for patients was 2.78 and 1.40 for controls ($p<0.001$). Multiple regression analysis demonstrated that: 1) DMFT index was associated with age, male sex, duration of mental illness, use of antidepressants, time since the last visit to the dentist, and snacking frequency; 2) community periodontal index was associated with male sex; and 3) plaque index was associated with age, male sex, education level, employment, monthly income, tooth brushing technique, and snacking frequency.

TREATMENT PLANS TO IMPROVE ORAL HEALTH OF PSYCHIATRIC INPATIENTS

Kisely (2011) suggested that at admission to hospital, nursing care plans should include an assessment of oral hygiene including the recording of factors that can affect oral health such as psychotropic medication and tobacco or substance use. Brief assessment tools such as the DFMT are available that can be completed by staff members. Toothbrushes and denture baths should be supplied to patients who should be instructed in their use. A study in Missouri demonstrated the efficacy of such programs, at least in terms of short-term improvements in oral hygiene (Almomani et al., 2006).

The greatest improvement in dental care for such patients likely is to occur by targeting people who report more problems with their teeth and dentures, including oral dyskinesias; those who have greater cognitive impairments, especially in executive function; and those who have diminished financial resources (Janardhanan et al., 2011).

ORAL HEALTH AND DENTAL NEEDS OF INSTITUTIONALIZED PSYCHIATRIC PATIENTS IN ISRAEL

According to the Dental Health Procedure no. 8.7 and Mental Health Procedure 65.002, version 3, updated on 26.10.2004, in Israel psychiatric patients with chronic mental disorders, hospitalized in psychiatric hospitals for over one year are entitled to dental care within the framework of mental health care services. A special fund was established in the Ministry of health to participate in financing these dental services. Careful use of the funds will ensure appropriate dental care for many hospitalized psychiatric patients. Dental Health Procedure 8.8 and Mental Health Procedure 65.003 from the same date delineate operational guidelines for dental clinics in psychiatric hospital settings. Procedures provide for dental care for all psychiatric inpatients with chronic illness and long term hospitalizations. However only five psychiatric hospitals have fully equipped dental clinics. In these five hospitals, in 2007, only 70% of inpatients had proper dental examination, 693 patients (45%) received dental treatment, and 506 of them received only emergency treatment. According to the procedures, hospitals that do not have dental clinics are responsible for providing dental care for long-term patients, in hospitals that have the appropriate facilities (Zusman et al., 2010).

THE REFORM OF PSYCHIATRIC SERVICES
IN ISRAEL AND DENTAL CARE

The Mental Health Rehabilitation Bill enacted in 2000 provides a basket of rehabilitation services, including dental care, for all mentally disabled individuals discharged from hospitals and living in the community. (Kraus, 2000) Dental care is provided by public and private clinics and paid for by the Ministry of Health. In 2007, a total of 1287 dental treatment plans were approved by the mental health rehabilitation committees (Massarwa, 2008); 766 psychiatric patients received dental treatment in the community at a total cost of 2.25 million New Shekels (NIS; approximately $450,000), that is NIS 3323 per patient (Zusman et al., 2010).

According to the 2011-1012 Report of dental treatment for mentally ill inpatients and for individuals with mental disorders who receive the basket of services in the community MOH (2013), in 2012 there were 1239 inpatients with chronic mental disorders, hospitalized for over one year, compared to 4499 such patients in 1996, a 75% reduction in 16 years. In 2012 there were 3616 inpatients during various hospitalization periods in mental health centers and in psychiatric departments in general hospitals. Of the 1239 patients hospitalized for over one year 951 were in the eight hospitals that have dental clinics. There were 288 inpatients in facilities without such services on the hospital grounds. Patients hospitalized for over one year are eligible for a free dental checkup, maintenance treatments, dental surgery and rehabilitative procedures. The yearly checkups and maintenance therapies are financed by the hospitals. The Ministry of Health covers the laboratory costs of rehabilitative treatments, x-rays, and materials in hospitals that have dental clinics. Hospitals without dental clinics are supposed to refer patients to clinics in other hospitals for treatment, or to provide ambulatory dental care on the hospital grounds. In such cases, the Ministry of Health covers the laboratory costs and 10% of the rehabilitative treatments, according to the price list of the Ministry.

In 2011-2012 there were 1374 dental checkups for psychiatric inpatients in the 8 mental health centers with dental clinics, i.e., checkups for 55% of the patients who were eligible for treatment. Of the 1374 patients examined, 800 applied for dental care (about 48%) and the rest of the patients refused treatment, despite repeated attempts by the dental clinic staff and psychiatric nurses to convince them of the necessity of treatment. In government hospitals, the dentists and oral hygienists supervised patients in proper oral hygiene and brushing. In the various departments, patients received tooth brushes and tooth paste, mouthwash, baking soda or agents based on chlorhexadine. Dental treatment included first aid, teeth cleaning, reconstruction, root canals, and tooth extractions. Of the 800 patients who applied for treatment in the 8 dental clinics, 243 completed maintenance therapy. In 2011-2012, 313 restorative dental treatments were approved, and 185 were completed (52%).

Zusman et al (2010) performed a systematic assessment of dental status and the oral health and dental needs of the chronically hospitalized psychiatric population in Israel. The survey, performed in fourteen psychiatric institutions (six government-owned and eight private), that provide care for 98% of all chronic psychiatric inpatients in Israel, was approved by the Ministry of Health's Institutional Review Board.

According to the Israel Ministry of Health (MOH) protocol, each hospitalized psychiatric patient is entitled to an annual dental check-up. In 2003, a random sample (20% of 1997 patients hospitalized longer than one year) was drawn from the MOH National Psychiatric Hospitalization Registry (NPHR). The dental examination was performed using a mirror and a probe, while the patient sat in front of a window under natural light. Patients in closed wards who were not mobile and elderly patients who were bedridden were examined in the wards. The DMFT index of overall dental status (number of decayed, missing or filled teeth in the permanent dentition) was calculated for each patient (Zusman et al., 2010).

Of the 254 inpatients that provided informed consent to be examined, 207 (81.5%) were free of soft tissue pathology. One person had a suspected malignancy and was referred to a medical centre for investigation. Leukoplakia was revealed in 14 cases, ulcerations in 13 cases (one connected to dentures), denture stomatitis in 5 cases, candidiasis in 2 cases, and abscess in 1 case. Other findings such aspigmentations were recorded in the 17 remaining cases (Zusman et al., 2010).

The 209 patients with schizophrenia had the highest mean DMFT score, 24.3±8.6, and the four patients with mood disorders had the lowest mean DMFT sore, 21.3±11.8. Schizophrenia patients also had the highest mean number caries, 2.8±4, and the highest mean number of missing teeth, 20±11.0 (Zusman et al., 2010).

This study revealed that chronic psychiatric inpatients in Israel generally suffer from poor oral health and urgently need guidance to promote oral health care, as well as treatment programs. Regardless of gender and age, psychiatric inpatients had a significantly higher mean number of both carious and missing teeth than the general population in Israel and other countries.

Though psychiatric patients with prolonged hospitalizations have high dental needs, their demand for treatment is low. Thus it is necessary to provide accessible dental treatment to patients with severe psychopathology who remain institutionalized and who are at increased risk of dental ill-health. For practical economic reasons, the earlier the treatment, the easier and less expensive it is. In the survey performed, 520 out of the total of almost 2000 inpatients (26%) needed prosthetic treatment. In the community, their treatment would cost 1.73 million New Israeli Shekels. As in many Western countries, following the implementation of the Mental Health Care Reform, many psychiatric inpatients were transferred to the community, and for these the Rehabilitation Act provides dental treatment and rehabilitation. Given that dental treatment offered during hospitalization is more cost-effective than similar treatment in the community, we believe that dental services should be accessible to all those entitled to it within hospital system, prior to discharge. The mobile oral health care unit introduced in the year 2000 that provides dental services to hospitals that do not have oral health care clinics is a step in that direction.

The findings of the present survey confirm the need to increase awareness of the importance of dental hygiene and oral health care, and to provide dental treatment for long-term psychiatric inpatients, including follow up care provided within the rehabilitation system, supported by law.

IMPROVEMENT IN ORAL AND DENTAL HEALTH OF PSYCHIATRIC INPATIENTS AFTER REORGANIZATION OF DENTAL SERVICES IN ISRAELI HOSPITALS

Following two large epidemiological surveys of oral health and care needs in hospitalized psychiatric patients performed in Israel in 1997 (Grinshpoon, 1997, 2003; Ramon et al., 2003), it was determined that there was an "urgent need for an intervention program to improve dental health care in chronic psychiatric inpatients" (Ramon et al., 2003).

Considerable collaborative efforts have since been made by the Division of Dental Health and Mental Health Services at the Israeli Ministry of Health to improve the existing dental services within the psychiatric inpatient system, including supplementation of the infrastructure and provision of dental equipment, increasing manpower in the existing clinics and establishing a central supervisory staff in the Division of Dental Health at the Ministry of Health. Regulations were implemented in the mental health services in the Ministry of Health requiring regular dental examinations and oral health care for every long-stay (>1 year) hospitalized inpatient. Hospitals that do not have dental clinics are required to outsource dental services. A special budgetary item was created for this purpose (Ramon et al., 2003). The Community-based Rehabilitation of the Mentally Disabled Act (2000) states that the state is responsible for funding dental treatments of mentally ill patients. An additional survey was performed in 2006 to assess effectiveness of this reorganization (Zussman et al., 2010).

Ponizovsky et al (2009) compared the data from these surveys to determine whether changes in dental health and oral care needs occurred between the two large cohorts representing psychiatric inpatient population before (1997) and after (2006) the reform of dental services in psychiatric hospitals in Israel. Significantly lower DMFT index and decayed component mean scores were found in the post-reform cohort compared with the pre-reform cohort. DMFT index mean scores were significantly lower for each, except the oldest age group, in the post- than in the pre-reform cohort. Likewise, decayed component was scored markedly lower in the post-reform cohort, except for the oldest age group, where this was significantly lower in the 1997 cohort ($t=8.56$, $p<.001$). In contrast, missing component scores were significantly higher in the post-reform cohort, excepting the youngest and the oldest age groups ($t=2.15$, $p<.05$ and $t=2.97$, $p<.01$, respectively). Filled component mean scores were significantly higher for the 18-34 and 55-64-year groups ($t=4.62$, $p<.001$ and $t=6.11$, $p<.001$, respectively) and lower for the 35-44-year group ($t=4.30$, $p<.001$) in the post- compared to the pre-reform cohort.

Independent of clinical diagnoses, all inpatients had lower scores on the DMFT decayed component in the post- than in the pre-reform cohort. For patients with diagnoses of schizophrenia and mood disorders (n=213), DMFT total mean scores were significantly lower in the post-reform cohort ($t=5.53$, $p<.001$ and $t=12.3$, $p<.001$, respectively). Mood disordered inpatients had a significantly higher score on the DMFT filled component ($t=4.20$, $p<.001$) and a significantly lower score on the DMFT missing component ($t=6.19$, $p<.001$) in the post-reform cohort, There were no between-cohort differences in the use and need for dentures.

Within the post-reform cohort, DMFT index and component mean scores in psychiatric inpatients 85 inpatients from hospitals that have a dental clinic and 169 patients from hospitals that use external dental services , both a significantly lower DMFT index and missing component scores (t=2.89, $p<.01$ and t=3.25, $p<.01$, respectively). Patients in hospitals with an on-site dental clinic had a higher filled permanent teeth score (t=2.84, $p<01$) than patients in hospitals with no dental clinic (Ponizovsky et al., 2009).

In Lev Hasharon Mental Health Center, Israel, for instance, there is an on-site dental clinic, and the nursing staff emphasizes the importance of oral hygiene in patient therapy groups. Great effort is invested in explanations and guidance for the promotion of optimal oral health care, and prevention of the development of caries. Various therapeutic techniques and methods are used to reduce anxiety related to dental treatments. Families are recruited to help convince the patients to receive appropriate dental treatment to maintain good oral hygiene. Despite these efforts, there is still a small stubborn group of patients that refused dental treatment (Rofe et al., 2010).

Following the reform the patients had less carious and missing teeth, and more treated teeth, and these findings were independent of gender and clinical diagnosis. The improved dental status of psychiatric inpatients following the reform is a result of the beneficial reorganization of dental services. Indeed, during this period fully equipped dental clinics were established in 10 of 18 psychiatric hospitals surveyed. In hospitals with on-site dental clinics that patients had meaningfully fewer missing teeth and more filled teeth than in hospitals that used external clinics. In addition, during that same period, there was intense deinstitutionalization and the Community-based Rehabilitation of the Mentally Disabled Act was introduced, and included integrated organizational framework to secure sufficient funding for the long-term rehabilitation for the mentally ill people. In addition, the Rehabilitation Law (2000) secured a special funding for dental care for those in the community. The reduction of inpatient beds along with a parallel growth of the number of community-based facilities created a situation where a substantial proportion of inpatients with better dental status and an urgent need for dental were transferred to community based services. Thus, the older inpatients with a relatively poorer oral status and a greater remained in hospital, and In this group DMF-T index and decayed component scores were significantly higher in the post-reform cohort compared to the pre-reform cohort. This finding suggests that the oldest inpatients who had poor dental health remained in hospitals during the post-reform period, and their younger and orally healthier counterparts were transferred from hospital to the community. Our finding is supported by a study demonstrating poor oral health and increased dental treatment needs among patients in psychiatric institutions for the elderly (Grinshpoon et al., 2006; Ponizovsky et al., 2009).

CONCLUSION

Nevertheless, we suggest that it is possible and important to contribute to the improvement of the oral health of psychiatric patients both in the hospital and in the community in the framework of improved quality of life for this population. Because, oral disease levels remain higher than in the general population, further steps are necessary to treat and prevent the progression of dental disorders. Owing to reluctance of many dentists to treat those with severe mental disorders, on-site dental service have proven to be the most effective venue for treatment and should be implemented in all mental health facilities. The allocation of funds for oral health care provided in the mental health care reform is a welcome step in the direction of improving oral health for individuals with chronic mental disorders, both in the hospital and in outpatient facilities.

REFERENCES

Almomani F, Brown C, Williams KB. The effect of an oral health promotion program for people with psychiatric disabilities. *Psychiatr Rehabil J* 2006; 29: 274-81.

Angelillo IF, Nobile GC, Pavia M, De Fazio P, Puca M, Amati A. Dental health and treatment needs in institutionalized psychiatric patients in Italy. *Community Dent Oral Epidemiol* 1995;23:360-364.

Bardow A, Nyvad B, Nauntofte B. Relationships between medication intake, complaints of dry mouth, salivary flow rate and composition, and the rate of tooth demineralization in situ. *Arch Oral Biol* 2001;46:413-423.

Community-Based Rehabilitation of the Mentally Disabled Act, Version no 2782. M/1506, July 2000 (in Hebrew).

Friedlander AH, Liberman RP. Oral health care for the patient with schizophrenia. *Spec Care Dentist* 1991;11:179-183.

Friedlander AH, Marder SR. The psychopathology, medical management and dental implications of schizophrenia. *J Am Dent Assoc* 2002;133:603-610.

Grinshpoon A. Evaluation of dental health services given to long-stay inpatients in governmental psychiatric hospitals and a proposal for an alternative model. Master's thesis, Ben-Gurion University of the Negev, Faculty of Health Sciences, Department of Health Systems Management, Israel, 1999.

Grinshpoon A, Zilber N, Lerner Y, Ponizovsky AM. Impact of a rehabilitation legislation on the survival in the community of long-term patients discharged from psychiatric hospitals in Israel. *Soc Psychiatry Psychiatr Epidemiol* 2006;41:87–94.

Grinshpoon A, Zusman SP, Weizman A, Ponizovsky AM. Dental health and the type of antipsychotic treatment: a study in schizophrenia patients. *Isr J Psychiatry Relat Sci* 2014 (in press).

Janardhanan T, Cohen CI, Kim S, Rizvi BF. Dental care and associated factors among older adults with schizophrenia. *J Am Dent Assoc* 2011;142:57-65.

Jovanovic S, Milovanovic SD, Gajic I, Mandic J, Latas M, Jankovic L. Oral health status of psychiatric in-patients in Serbia and implications for their dental care. *Croat Med J* 2010;51:443-450.

Jyoti B, Muneeshwar PD, Srivastava R, Singh AR, Kiran M, Simlai J. Oral helath status in treatment needs of psychiatric inpatients in Ranchi, India. *J Indian Acad Oral Med Radiol* 2012;24:177-181.

Kisely S, Quek LH, Pais J, Lalloo R, Johnson NW, Lawrence D. Advanced dental disease in people with severe mental illness: systematic review and meta-analysis. *Br J Psychiatry* 2011;199:187–193.

Kraus, Boaz. Legal Codex for Health Issues: Mentally Ill, Protected, Incompetent, The Law. Ozar Hamishpat, Netanya, 2000 (in Hebrew).

Kumar M, Chandu GN, Shafiulla MD. Oral health status and treatment needs in institutionalized psychiatric patients: One year descriptive cross sectional study. *Indian J Dent Res* 2006;17:171–177.

Li X, Kolltveit KM, Tronstad L, Olsen I. Systemic diseases caused by oral infection. *Clin Microbiol Rev* 2000;13:547-558.

Massarwa A-S. Dental treatment to psychiatric patients in psychiatric hospitals and to entitled to rehabilitation basket, Annualreport 2007. Ministry of Health, 2008 (in Hebrew).

McCreadie RG, Stevens H, Henderson J, Hall D, McCaul R, Filik R, etal. The dental health of people with schizophrenia. *Acta Psychiatr Scand* 2004;110:306-310.

Ministry of Health, Department of Dental Services, Annual Report, 2011-2012, Jerusalem, 2013.

Mirza I, Day R, Phelan M, Sulff-Cochrane V. Oral health of psychiatric in patients- A point prevalence survey of intercity hospital. *Psychiatr Bull* 2001;25:143–145.

Page MM. Psychotropic drugs and dentistry. *Aust Prescriber* 2007; 30:98-101.

Ponizovsky AM, Zusman SP, Dekel D, Masarwa AE, Ramon T, Natapov L, Yoffe R, Weizman A, Grinshpoon A. Effect of implementing dental services in Israeli psychiatric hospitals on the oral and dental health of inpatients. *Psychiatr Serv* 2009;60:799-803.

Ramon T, Grinshpoon A, Zusman SP, Weizman A. Oral health and treatment needs of institutionalized chronic psychiatric patients in Israel. *Eur Psychiatry* 2003;18:101-105.

Rekha R, Hiremath SS, Bharath S. Oral health status and treatment requirements of hospitalized psychiatric patients in Bangalore City: A comparative study. *J Indian Soc Pedod Prev Dent* 2002;20:63–67.

Rofe Z, Behrbalk P, Bleich A, Melamed Y. Oral hygiene among patients with chronic mental disorders. The Medical 14/7/2010 (in Hebrew). (http://www.themedical.co.il/Article.aspx?medicalField=17&itemID= 2955).

Shah VR, Priyadarshini J, Patel N. Oral health of psychiatric patients: A cross-sectional comparision study *Dent Res J* (Isfahan) 2012; 9:209–214.

Shukla GD, Shrivastava RP. A psychiatric study of cases attending dental OPD of a teaching general hospital, Jhansi. *Indian J Psychiatry* 1983;25:198–202.Tang WK, sun FCS, ungvari GS, O'donell D. Oral Health of Psychiatric in patients in Hong Kong. *Int J Soc Psychiatry* 2004;50:186–191.

Tani H, Uchida H, Suzuki T, Shibuya Y, Shimanuki H, Watanabe K, Den, R., Nishimoto, M., Hirano, J., Takeuchi, H., Nio, S., Nakajima, S., Kitahata R, Tsuboi T, Tsunoda K, Kikuchi T, Mimura M. Dental conditions in inpatients with schizophrenia: a large-scale multi-site survey. *BMC Oral Health* 2012;12: 32.

Zusman SP, Ponizovsky AM, Dekel D, Masarwa AE, Ramon T, Natapov L, Grinshpoon A. An assessment of the dental health of chronic institutionalized patients with psychiatric disease in Israel. *Spec Care Dentist* 2010;30:18-22.

WHAT IS THE CONTRIBUTION OF THE BOOK?

Patients with mental disorders have needs in common with healthy people in addition to their own specific needs. However, the frequency of unmet needs varies substantially across need domains and there is a major gap between a need for help and the actual help received from mental health services. This gap results from the obvious discrepancies in the assessments of needs by staff, caregivers and by the patients themselves. Hence, negotiation of the different evaluation perspectives is a robust approach to addressing the specific needs of our patients.

Further, we described the psychiatric services that currently exist in Israel and provided examples of supported education and employment programs for individuals with severe mental illness that illustrate how their needs can be fulfilled within the rehabilitation framework. As Israel underwent the reform of psychiatric hospitalization services, we described some benefits of the changes, which enabled patients with mental health disabilities that were hospitalized in psychiatric institutions for long periods of time to relocate to the community. We also addressed issues of new institutionalization in the community.

The impact of how the ethnic background of patients who attended mental health services for the first time brought about substantial variation in the rates of detection of emotional distress and psychopathological symptoms is discussed. This variation was meaningfully associated with lower sense of self-efficacy and perceived social support among Israeli Arabs, as compared to Israeli Jews. Together with lack of knowledge about and negative attitudes to mental disorders and treatment, these feelings led to a longer treatment lag among this minority group. Because these factors are potentially modifiable, educational programs tailored to the different consumer sectors and the different community gatekeepers of access to psychiatric care are needed. Programs designed to raise confidence in the treatability of mental disorders and to shorten treatment lag need to be implemented.

We now know that in general, the Israeli population affected by terrorism does not perceive their mental and social suffering as requiring specialized interventions. Israelis who experience ongoing terrorism and threats of war, have a high level of social resilience. The consequences of this "invulnerability" might be a potential increase of public levels of aggressiveness and rise of violent crime that warrant further investigation.

The need for emergency psychiatric services in Israel is presented. These developing services might play a preventive role by enabling the early detection of mental illness, preventing deterioration and consequent psychiatric hospitalization. Another function of these services, in the case of pre-existing mental disorders, is to enhance the awareness of mental disorders and offer family members an opportunity to encourage patients to improve cooperation with available services and treatment.

We have familiarized our readers with mental health legislation and mental health services that address the needs and rights of individuals with mental disorders while protecting the safety and security of society as a whole.

Finally, the example of oral health services illustrates the needs of mentally disabled people for medical non-psychiatric services. We showed the benefits of the implementation of dental health services in the mental health system in Israel. The improvement of the oral health of psychiatric patients both in the hospital and in the community contributes to better physical health and quality of life of individuals with mental impairments. Despite unequivocal success in this field, oral disease levels in our patients remain higher than in the general population. Hence, further steps are necessary to not only treat but mainly prevent the progression of dental disorders. Allocation of funds for oral health care provided in the mental health care reform is necessary for individuals with chronic mental disorders, both in the hospital and in outpatient facilities.

We hope that the knowledge concentrated in this book will serve as an example to benefit not only local but also international mental health professionals who seek to address the needs of patients with mental disorders and disabilities.

ABOUT THE AUTHORS

Alexander M. Ponizovsky, M.D., Ph.D. is an internationally recognized researcher in the field of psychiatry. His areas of expertise include schizophrenia; suicidal behavior; addiction; hospital and community-based mental health and rehabilitation services; evaluation for different treatment programs with regard to quality of life and psychosocial outcomes assessment; psychological distress and psychosocial resources, maintenance treatment; migration and mental health, and attachment research in psychopathology. Dr. Ponizovsky earned his M.D. degree at the Moscow Medical Academy and his Ph.D. at the Moscow Psychiatric Research Institute and Bekhterev's Psycho-neurological Research Institute, St. Petersburg, Russia. After immigration to Israel in 1991, he was awarded the KAMEA fellowship established by the Israeli Ministry Immigrant Absorption for distinguished immigrant scientists.

Currently, Dr. Ponizovsky is the KAMEA Professor of Psychiatry and Advisor on Mental Health Research in the Department of Mental Health Services at the Israeli Ministry of Health. Dr. Ponizovsky has more than 150 scientific publications, including 10 chapters in international collections. He has lectured at many research meetings and conferences. He is a member of the editorial board and reviewer for more than 60 medical journals. Dr. Ponizovsky is the recipient of several grants from the Israeli Ministry of Science, Zionist Forum of Soviet Jews and for his research on *Epidemiology of Suicide ideation in an Immigrant Population*. He is also the recipient of international awards, including the International Lifetime Achievement Award for outstanding contributions to Medicine and Healthcare. Dr. Ponizovsky is listed in *Who's Who in Science and Engineering*.

Alexander Grinshpoon, M.D., M.H.A., PH.D., is Director of Sha'ar Menashe Mental Health Center, Hadera, Israel and Clinical Associate Professor at the Rappaport Faculty of Medicine, Technion, Israel Institute of Technology, Haifa, Israel. He served as Director of Mental Health Services in the Israel Ministry of Health from 2001 to 2006. He former positions include Director of Tirat Carmel Mental Health Center, and Head of the Department of Psychiatry in the Israel Defense Forces, and Director of the Reservists Section of the Central Mental Health Clinic for the Israel Defense Forces.

The structural reform of Mental Health Services in Israel was implemented during Dr. Grinshpoon's administration of the Mental Health Services in the Ministry of Health. The number of inpatient beds was reduced by more than fifty percent. The Law for Rehabilitation of the Mentally Handicapped in the Community was initiated and the community based services for individuals with mental disorders significantly increased by over one thousand percent. During that period, the Ministry of Health participated in a multi-national study "From Epidemiology to Mental Health Action", the results of which are included in this book.

Prof. Grinshpoon earned his MD degree at Kishinev State University, Faculty of Medicine, USSR, and his Master's in Health Administration and PhD in Medical Management at Ben-Gurion University, Beersheba, Israel. He is currently the President of the Northern Branch of the Israel Psychiatric Association, and Head of the Law Committee of the Israel Psychiatric Association. Prof. Grinshpoon has received research grants from the Ministry of Health Social Affairs, Ministry of Finance, as well as from the Israel Anti-Drug Committee, and pharmaceutical companies. He has presented the results of his research at scientific conferences in Israel and abroad.

Prof. Grinshpoon has published over one hundred articles in international scientific journals, and serves as reviewer for leading journals in the field of psychiatry. He is currently the head of the only fellowship program in forensic psychiatry in Israel. The book, Forensic Psychiatry in Israel (Hebrew), co-authored by Prof. Grinshpoon is a nationally acclaimed textbook in all academic libraries in Israel.

INDEX

G

H

Q

R

S

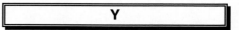
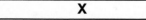